Further Praise for

Transforming the Nature of Health

"A fascinating journey to move from dis-ease to well-being, from aloneness and separation to community and oneness. Marcey Shapiro looks with new eyes at the organisms that share 'our' bodies, proposing a model of peace in the realm of medicine and within each of us. She advocates a different understanding of illness. Illustrated with intriguing stories from her clinical practice, where she uses tools of conventional medicine, science, and natural approaches, this is a refreshing read that contains profound insights and a deep spiritual message. *Transforming the Nature of Health* is sprinkled with very practical meditations and easy-to-follow advice that will change the way you think. A must-read for anyone dealing with a body that is out of balance either physically or emotionally."

—CAROL SABICK DE LA HERRAN,
executive director and president of The Monroe Institute

"Marcey Shapiro articulates the perfect prescription for better health: focus on positive energy, forgiveness, and love and where appropriate utilize new technologies and therapies that harmonize with nature to restore balance in our bodies and our lives. She challenges the conventional thinking of modern medicine and invites a new perspective that will help transform health and health care."

—HELEN GRACIE, cofounder of Scenar Health

Transforming

THE NATURE OF

Health

A Holistic Vision of Healing
That Honors Our Connection
to the Earth, Others, and Ourselves

Marcey Shapiro, MD
Foreword by Robert Golden, MD

North Atlantic Books
Berkeley, California

Published by
North Atlantic Books   Cover photo by Susan Quasha
P.O. Box 12327   Cover and book design by Susan Quasha
Berkeley, California 94712   Printed in the United States of America

Transforming the Nature of Health: A Holistic Vision of Healing That Honors Our Connection to the Earth, Others, and Ourselves is sponsored by the Society for the Study of Native Arts and Sciences, a nonprofit educational corporation whose goals are to develop an educational and cross-cultural perspective linking various scientific, social, and artistic fields; to nurture a holistic view of arts, sciences, humanities, and healing; and to publish and distribute literature on the relationship of mind, body, and nature.

North Atlantic Books' publications are available through most bookstores. For further information, visit our website at www.northatlanticbooks.com or call 800-733-3000.

MEDICAL DISCLAIMER: The following information is intended for general information purposes only. Individuals should always see their health care provider before administering any suggestions made in this book. Any application of the material set forth in the following pages is at the reader's discretion and is his or her sole responsibility.

Library of Congress Cataloging-in-Publication Data

Shapiro, Marcey, 1957–
Transforming the nature of health : a holistic vision of healing that honors our connection to the Earth, others, and ourselves / Marcey Shapiro.
     p. cm.
Includes index.
Summary: "Countering conventional medicine's view of health care as a protracted war with germs and disease, *Transforming the Nature of Health* asks us to consider what medicine would look like if we were at peace with nature and offers a fresh and often playful understanding of health and connectedness based on love, meaning, and respect"—Provided by publisher.
ISBN 978-1-58394-361-8
1. Harmony (Philosophy) 2. Health—Religious aspects. 3. Love. 4. Spiritual life. 5. Consciousness. I. Title.
B105.H37S53 2011
128—dc23
                              2011018464
1 2 3 4 5 6 7 8 9 UNITED 17 16 15 14 13 12

*For love, and a life journey of living from the Heart,
with all its mystery and wonder.*

Author's Note:

I DISCUSS MANY PATIENTS' EXPERIENCES THROUGHOUT the book. To protect their privacy, the names of my patients and certain identifying details of their cases have been altered, though the essence of their experiences has been preserved.

Contents

Foreword

ROBERT GOLDEN, MD

A s a Western-trained surgical sub-specialist, my entire medi-cal career has been framed by linear thinking, surgical decision-making, "fixing" problems, and separating the physical body from the spiritual being. I was in a box—my patients came to me with a physi-cal problem, I diagnosed the disorder, offered therapy to eliminate the complaint, and the encounter was over. Done deal. For twenty-five years, I rationalized my practice of medicine to exclude the spirit of the individual and to disregard all the internal and environmental fac-tors that prompted the patient to enter my office with a complaint. I somehow thought this was the right way to be a healer.

Over the past several years, my partner and I have been on an increasingly deep spiritual journey … exploring meaning, mind-body connection, vibrational alignment, purpose, love, source, being. As I opened to this connection, the universe instilled clarity into my life: we are physical manifestations of spiritual source energy.

I first met Marcey Shapiro at an Abraham-Hicks Tahiti cruise workshop. Immediately, her energy was palpable and soothing. There was a deep connection. Soon I discovered that she is a Western-trained medical doctor (MD) practicing a very unusual blend of care. Her interests vary from classic Western medicine to acupuncture, en-ergy work, homeopathic remedies, and so much more. As Marcey and I became friends, I saw and felt a compassionate, aware, and generous total physician. At her core is a person of love, the source of her heal-ing powers.

Marcey Shapiro's perspective in *Transforming the Nature of Health* is so much more than an epiphany. She drills deep into philosophy, religious traditions, politics, physics, and biology with passion, humor, and integrity. As I got lost in this enlightenment, the veil of Western thinking was lifted. Clearly, a patient visiting me with a physical complaint had traveled far down the road of non-alignment, sometimes for years. The physical manifestation of discord with truth and contentment grows and torments the soul until we wake up and pay attention to our heart.

Marcey writes this book from her heart. She clearly visualizes truth with complete non-judgment. I came to tears with her description of the tortured stories of her patients. She then gently redirects the focus to positivity and alignment with total acceptance, love, and wisdom. There is no attachment to the outcome … a patient may decide to just stay where they are, and yet, love remains the mainstay of the encounter.

My specialty is urology, a surgical sub-specialty involving linear thinking, judgment, and outcomes. I've practiced for more than thirty years. As I became more aware of the healing art of medicine, Marcey showed up and I was able to visualize, through her, infinite possibilities in the marriage of surgeon and holistic urologist. Marcey honors the "doctor-patient relationship" and clearly practices the art of allowing while counseling and advising her patients. And she does this without judgment. Without her even knowing or certainly taking any credit, she has guided me onto a different path of healer, that of exploring solutions on the basis of love. I am so grateful for Marcey Shapiro.

Transforming the Nature of Health has changed the core of my practice. Whereas before I looked for a physical explanation for a symptom complex, I now search for the spiritual link. Fear, anger, resentment, lack of self-worth, and guilt are the likely culprits. There is so much more. We are connected, one organism on Mother Earth taking care of each other in loving kindness. This is the epiphany I received from Marcey. Our positive energy and focus, our thoughts attracting our wants, our ability to heal ourselves without guilt, only hope. Enjoy.

Introduction

A new scientific truth does not triumph by convincing its
opponents and making them see the light, but rather because its opponents eventually die, and a new generation
grows up that is familiar with it.
—MAX PLANCK, *physicist, inventor of quantum theory,*
Nobel Prize winner 1918

I HAVE BEEN ENTHRALLED BY TINY life forms since I first peeked into a
"Junior Scientist" microscope when I was eight years old. There, I
discovered an unseen world, as vast and diverse as any terrain visible on
the surface of the planet. I found myself fascinated by the presence of
an abounding universe, infinitely complex and textured but impercep-
tible to the naked eye. A few years later I was captivated by the same
sense of wonder as I gazed upon the vast cosmos through the lens of
the telescope. The identical allure has magnetized me toward exploration of mystical realms, invisible through any lens except the heart.

As a child, I imagined that everything including microorganisms
had human interactions and personalities. The vast numbers and
grand diversity of the microscopic world fascinated me. Through the
tiny aperture of the lens, I saw thousands of little beings: rotifers,
euglenas, paramecia, and others, teeming in a mere drop of pond water. Different, equally fascinating organisms thrived in a bit of my
saliva. I made up fanciful stories about them and wondered what they
were doing in their little communities. Do some bacteria like other
bacteria? Do they have needs, desires, and friendships? Although I did
not get any specific verbal answers, this line of questioning always led
me to friendly and positive feelings. Growing up with free access to
nature, I developed a confidence in the kindness and intelligence of
the natural world.

In biological medicine, on the other hand, microorganisms are generally reviled, despite a growing understanding of the importance of "healthy probiotic bacteria," especially those of the intestinal tract. Fear of microorganisms never sat well with me, so the idea that started this book was the simple question, "Could there be another way, biomedically, to understand and relate to microscopic life?" Of course, I already suspected what answers would come, as I have experienced and worked with the natural world in a participatory and cooperative manner my entire life.

When I began this book, I did not realize the direction it would take, and how medicine, biology, quantum theory and mechanics, mystical insights, ecology, resilience theory, and channeling might all neatly dovetail. I started *Transforming the Nature of Health* merely as an attempt to revisit our relationship with the world of microscopic organisms. But as I looked at the complexities of human relationships with microorganisms, I quickly saw a correspondence between the microcosm of our treatment of miniscule life forms and the macrocosm of human relationships. How we treat and relate to "them" is how we think about others, nature, and ourselves.

Metamorphosis of our relationship with microorganisms is one facet of the great transformation of our understanding of the universe that is currently transpiring. We are, as a global civilization, beginning to realize that consciousness itself is the great creative force of all life. We are starting to appreciate the dizzying wisdom that the external world always reflects the inner world. We have a dawning of understanding that all of humanity is connected. These are fundamental and profound insights that spiritual teachers from diverse traditions have shared throughout the ages. Today cutting-edge science is proving the "reality" of these ancient mystical truths. Every branch of science and spirituality is affected by this new comprehension. Yet as a global civilization, we barely understand the enormous ramifications of the changes that are upon us.

We are spiritual beings engaged in a physical existence. We remain spiritual beings throughout every moment of our lives. Most people believe in an underlying spiritual reality greater than our physical existence. So it is odd that as a society we still agree with the conclusions of a "science" that historically rejects and ignores this reality. It is ironic indeed that it is precisely the leading edges of our very materialistic science establishment that lead us back to what we already know in our hearts: the underlying unity of all being.

The current shift is at least as profound as the one that must have been felt in the fourth century BC when observers realized that the Earth is round rather than flat. It is as immense as that which occurred when Galileo provided astronomical evidence to support Copernicus's observations that our planet is one of several that revolve around the sun, thus proving that Earth is not the center of the universe. Heretical as each of these notions was in its day, they were, of course, a more correct understanding of the physical Earth and celestial mechanics.

Galileo's observations did not serve the dominant powers of his generation and eventually undermined much of their doctrine. In one generation, European civilization's entire understanding of the world was altered. It is now obvious to us that the Earth revolves around the sun, and that most of the stars we see are suns, and that the stars in our galaxy all revolve around something else: the galactic core.

There are parallel shockwaves upon us now, inaugurated by the convergence of similarities between long-held spiritual wisdom teachings about the nature of reality and the observations of cutting-edge science. A big part of this shockwave currently emanates from the field of physics. It was initiated by Max Planck and elaborated by twentieth-century luminaries of quantum physics including Albert Einstein, Niels Bohr, Werner Heisenberg, Eugene Wigner, Erwin Schrödinger, Louis de Broglie, and Wolfgang Pauli.

In the late nineteenth century physics was viewed as a virtually complete field of science. Max Planck, a father of quantum theory, was discouraged by his physics professor, Philipp von Jolly, from pursuing a career in the study of physics, as von Jolly believed that "in this field, almost everything is already discovered, and all that remains is to fill a few holes."[1] But in the last one hundred years, a new world of startling and inspiring research has come from the previously sleepy domain of physics through the discovery and examination of the quantum world.

The reverberations of quantum mechanics, an offering from the heart of "hard" science, have implications for our understanding of the very nature of physical reality. Quantum theory brings us to another rung of an endless evolutionary spiral, to a perception of the natural world that is more in line with traditional spiritual and mystical insights from worldwide traditions than is the old mechanistic science. New sciences are developing that take our expanded understanding of the universe into account. These result in societal shifts as the old "flat Earth" paradigm fades away and a comprehension of the implications of our interconnection is born.

Ecology is also in the forefront in informing the shift of understanding. When looking at complex systems such as the ecosystem of a wetland or an intestinal tract, we find that balance, cooperation, and diversity rather than competition or "survival of the fittest" are the actual means to promotion of health and well-being. A related and growing area of scientific discourse studies resilience in various systems. Resilience, whether in agriculture, economics, or human and animal health, depends upon a balance among multiple complex interacting factors. Resilience in systems demonstrates that reductionism, the preferred method of scientific discourse for the last two hundred-odd years, is an antiquated and obsolete model for understanding living systems.

Why? Because reductionism looks at one or two isolated factors and from those attempts to determine meaningful information about the whole. Usually these individual components to be studied are isolated from their environment. If they were living or part of living systems, they are usually killed or dead for science to study them. We are now experiencing the limitations of that approach as super-infections multiply, bee and pollinator colonies collapse worldwide, and formerly rich and vast biodiverse regions like the Great Plains become chemical-sodden dust bowls. We have missed the forest for the color of the twigs upon one branch of one tree.

Reductionist science is akin to taking a bird wing, chopping it up in a blender and isolating the constituent proteins, then analyzing one or two proteins to study in more detail in order to determine information about mechanisms of flight. This method is slow, cumbersome, and roundabout, and it ultimately yields little useful information. A child flapping her arms is probably on a more productive track. Still, many scientists could and do devote their entire lives to this type of dissection. But we are seeing that in reality the whole is greater than the sum of its parts, and no matter how many isolated parts we study, we eventually find that entire systems flourish only in the interaction of many, many fluctuating factors. A bird flies not because it has this type of collagen, or that shape of bone. Some birds have large wings, others small ones; some, like ducks and geese, store a lot of body fat, while others like hummingbirds store relatively little. Some birds are social and will fly only in interaction. Some birds are so shy, we presume they fly but no one has ever seen them do so.

We are learning that living systems must be studied as a whole, complete with all their messy interactions. And though it might seem intuitively obvious, we are just now learning that thriving living systems are best studied while they remain alive, intact, and vibrant. We are just now developing tools to look at this complexity. These tools, hidden in plain sight, are provided by observation of the harmonious interactions of the natural world. Nature is self-organizing and infinitely creative, exhibiting great intelligence and wisdom.

Western medicine, despite all its technological dazzle, has until recently remained staunchly mired in the old paradigms. This too is changing, in the gentle way that Planck discussed in the quote that opens this section of the book. New ways of thinking are emerging and the young are used to them, thinking of them as normal, and the old inflexible folks are dying out. Science advances, as Planck quipped, "one funeral at a time." We are learning more about the web of interaction and the value of honoring the whole. We are in the process of observing the birth of a quantum understanding of human biology. These understandings will result in a radical transformation of our conceptions of health and disease.

The outgoing medical perspective of illness is that it is a disease of body or mind that seems to happen from outside our participation and is certainly outside our desires. In biomedicine we do not treat or try to correct the cause of most illness. We believe disease is an abnormal process that is set in motion by external factors such as environmental toxins, random accidents and mishaps, noxious influence of various organisms like bacteria or viruses, or uncontrollable internal circumstances such as our genetic make-up. Because these are largely elements we cannot control, we feel vulnerable, fearful, and disempowered regarding our health. The belief that the locus of control of one's physical body is outside us leads to a deep sense of anxiety.

Disease is thought of as random and capricious, though we do acknowledge some "risk factors." For example, smoking is generally accepted as a prominent risk factor for lung cancer. It is of interest, though, that most people who smoke do not get lung cancer. There certainly have been few if any studies examining the differences in health outcomes, for example, between smokers of organically grown loose tobacco and the majority of people who smoke processed commercial cigarettes. Is it the tobacco itself that increases the risk of cancer, or the act of smoking, or could it be chemical additives in the cigarettes or something else? Commercial cigarettes contain hundreds of questionable additives. In 1994 a list of 599 "approved" additives was released by six major cigarette manufacturers.[2] Moreover, commercial cigarettes are a surprising but notorious source of toxic radiation exposure. This fact is acknowledged by the U.S. Environmental Protection Agency.[3] I'm not trying to argue for smoking here. I am merely trying to demonstrate some of the complexity inherent even in a widely acknowledged risk.

Most of our attempts at prevention of disease devolve to analysis of confusing and partisan debate about risk factors. But we rarely agree on an understanding of even a simple risk. The end result for health care consumers is more feelings of befuddlement and disempowerment.

Contemporary medicine grudgingly acknowledges the ramifications of lifestyle factors and personal choices upon health. But very few practitioners and fewer researchers admit or even believe that thoughts, mind, focus, and consciousness are the most important determinants of health. This is changing. Tiny microbes may come to have an enormous role in shifting our perceptions.

Restructuring our relationship with the microscopic world and other beings that have been ignored or reviled has profound implications for our worldview. It requires us to truly embrace an expanded understanding of life and consciousness, one that includes everyone and every thing. Not only every human—it means revisiting our entire relationship with the natural world. A system shift toward true health means acknowledging that everyone, even people we dislike, has a valuable place and purpose. We are all related and every interaction is meaningful. This understanding fundamentally changes how we see individual health and the health care system.

I wrote *Transforming the Nature of Health* from this new perspective. I asked nature questions about interrelationship, and observed the answers that came to me. I learned in multitudinous ways: from the patients who visited my office, the links that people sent me on various social media, books that inspired me, cutting-edge scientific research, science fiction, long walks in nature, and my own meditations. I asked if there might be a different set of premises that we could employ which might lead us to more harmonious and cohesive conclusions about the nature of health and healing.

This volume, part dream, part new science, part memoir, and part philosophical treatise, is one fruit of my dialogue with nature. It is an offering of hope, and a vision for a different type of cultural and societal understanding of health with a new view of the possible role of medicine and healing. The responses of nature to my questions are characterized by a dramatically different, more loving, and more accurate set of answers than those offered by the "modern" biological sciences. They are much more in line with the answers hinted at by systems theory, sacred texts, and quantum mechanics.

Transforming the Nature of Health, though referencing science, invites readers on a deeply personal journey. This is consistent with spiritual insights and new physics, both of which demonstrate that the observer influences and becomes a part of the observation. So my book, of necessity, has to do with all of who I am—my personal experience of the natural world, my experiences of medical training and medical practice, and my mystical explorations.

Throughout the book, the question of "what is health and what is illness?" is reconsidered. Our responses to health and illness are examined, and prevailing cultural beliefs about the causes and meaning of illness are re-evaluated. The role of microorganisms in this discussion is reframed, as are supposedly abnormal cellular and organ processes like cancer and inflammation. *Transforming the Nature of Health* is written from a perspective that is uniquely inclusive of the consciousness of the natural world. In this model, the world is not dead matter to be acted upon. Nor are we passive victims, subject to random and capricious disease processes.

Instead, in this understanding the world, all of physical matter, is our collective vision. It is an ever-evolving manifestation of our beliefs, desires, expectations, and experimentation. We are participants and creators, bound by our creations only until we create anew. From this perspective illness is something vastly different from how it is viewed biomedically.

We are in the midst of a momentous awakening, a transformation of consciousness that embraces this awareness. Nobel Laureate in physics Eugene Wigner summed up discoveries in twentieth-century quantum physics with this amazing observation: "It will remain remarkable, in whatever way our future concepts may develop, that the very study of the external world led to the scientific conclusion that the content of the consciousness is the ultimate universal reality."[4]

So, ultimately, *Transforming the Nature of Health* is an invitation to imagine together the role of healing in a world that understands that divine Love is the underlying substance that makes up physical reality. Woven within and through this remains the original inspiration of kindness toward all beings: insects, plants, animals, and even microorganisms. I welcome you to join me in exploring our magnificent world of love, health, and meaning.

—CHAPTER ONE—

The Heart of the Matter

THE HEART OF A HUMAN embryo is one of the first recognizable structures formed. The embryo is initially a flat pancake-like grouping of three layers of cells: endoderm, ectoderm, and mesoderm. These layers give rise to all the tissues of the body.

The cardiovascular system begins to develop early on, while the embryo is still flat. The heart arises from the center of these layers, the mesoderm.[1] The area that will become the heart is called the cardiogenic region. It begins to form in the third week of fetal development. By day 22 the heart is "spontaneously" beating.

The scientific answer that this occurs "spontaneously" is not very satisfying, because it is clearly not happenstance. The timing is exact. Nature clearly sees the establishment of a beating heart as an essential initial step that occurs as part of an exquisitely ordered sequence in the generation of life. It is important to note that the heart is not necessary to provide biochemical nutrients for the tiny embryo. In its first two weeks the embryo receives its nourishment from the yolk sac. After implantation in the uterine wall, the placenta forms, and fetal circulation and nutrient delivery, especially early on, is entirely dependent upon the mother. And when the heart begins to beat, at day 22, it does not yet have chambers or a circulatory system into which it could pump blood. So why is the tiny beating heart of the three-week-old embryo so important to the project of life? Could it be that the beating heart provides a different, but still essential, type of nourishment?

By acknowledging an underlying spiritual non-physical reality, it is easier to see what is happening during early fetal development. The heart is physically and metaphorically the direct pathway to and from the inner being. Most of us already understand or trust that there is a sacred magic in this primary process. Perhaps what actually happens is the heart begins to beat in response to an impulse originating from the infinite reservoir of life-force. The beating heart is a link, at our core, between the physical and the non-physical, resonating to the rhythms of both. The heartbeat arises in a minute flat cluster of cells to resound in tune with great cosmic forces that organize physical life.

The heart begins to beat so early on because it is central to the project of physical life. The heart exists to bathe each of us, through-out our lives—each tiny developing human, each child, and each full-grown adult—in our own unique electromagnetic field. Each heart beats its particular vibrational tune in resonance with the drum of a greater non-physical rhythm. What does this mean? It is well known that if you pluck one stringed instrument in a room or tap a drum, others nearby will vibrate as well. If there are several instruments in the vicinity, each reverberates in resonant harmony to the original tone. Yet none of the sounds produced by differing instruments are identical, though they technically play the same tone. The "body" of each instrument determines the depth, richness, and complexity of the note each sounds. The type of wood and the age and skill of the crafter who created it are among the many factors that conjoin to cre-ate each instrument's unique sound.

It is the same with us. We are each unique instruments of the di-vine. We each produce a symphony of vibrational tones. One's heart, mediating between physical and non-physical, is the pivotal instru-ment upon which the concert of each physical life is played. It trans-lates and transmits the transcendent into each person's life path. Our hearts reverberate the voice of the divine because they are always connected to it.

Our heart creates the strongest electromagnetic field of our body. It is up to sixty times as strong as the field the brain generates and can be detected up to fifteen feet from the body.[2] This means that it plays the loudest and clearest tones of any tissue. Our cells, organs, and mind can clearly resonate. The personal heart field affects not only oneself but others as well.[3] The more harmoniously our heart resonates with our inner divinity, as demonstrated by peacefulness and coherence, the greater the amplitude of field it generates. This effect has been measured in laboratories.[4]

There are rhythms of life all around us, suffusing material reality, observable in great and small tidal forces. Perhaps "modern" scientists have not discovered them because none were seeking that type of information. However, osteopaths, craniosacral practitioners, acupuncturists, Qi nei tsang practitioners, and others involved with bio-energetic healing modalities attune themselves with ease to various broader pulsations. Some of these are electromagnetic, but others, while easily perceived, are sensed in the bio-energetic field, and we currently have no tools or instruments to measure them.

Remember the old adage, "If your only tool is a hammer, you will always be looking only for nails." Science not rooted in any broader context does not seek knowledge of the link between our bodies and our inner being, or evidence of continuity between physical and non-physical reality. In fact, it studiously avoids looking at those particular elephants in the living room. Even if scientists stumble upon such information, results are usually discounted, explained away, or ignored. This is not an accident, and in Chapter Seven, "Maps of the Worlds," I'll explain more about how the separation of science and spirit happened.

At the heart of us, a physiologic connection exists between our divinity and our physical existence. I propose that life force itself animates the heart, and that is why the heart must beat so early on. It is also why the heart is intuitively so sacred to us. Notice how many Catholic churches called "Sacred Heart" are scattered around the Earth.

Could science find this connection? Of course it could, if it were a type of science that was pursuing this information. It is not especially difficult to learn to feel the pulsations of life force with one's hands. Anyone who has the desire to develop the sensitivity can do so, with practice. Acupuncturists feel it in the flow of Qi. Cranial osteopaths and craniosacral practitioners learn to feel the breath of life in the tissues. Even materialistic science is aware that our human hands are sensitive to motion measured in microns. Think of how easy it is to feel the slightest breeze on your skin.

Let's look further into embryological development and consider what it might indicate if we know ourselves as spiritual beings in physical form. The drama of embryologic life continues with the development of the head and the brain. The formation of the brain gives more credence to a comprehension that the heart is the "heart of the matter," rather than the brain.

Brain development begins in the fifth week after conception, and early brain activity is noted in the sixth week. When the embryo becomes a three-dimensional being rather than a flat collection of tissues, the area around the heart folds. The nucleus of the cellular material that eventually becomes our brain is contained in the folded area, just above the heart. So when we are tiny embryos, our heart and brain are essentially connected structures. In early brain development, these tissues separate, and the portion of tissue that will become the brain begins to unfold and lift upward. The heart moves downward (caudally), settling in the neck region for a while before finally locating itself in the chest.

It is amazing that the cells that shape and comprise our brain literally form from the tissue closest to the beating heart! Because the brain arises with the heart, the two are intimately connected through various nerve pathways and remain so throughout a person's life. There are more neuronal connections leading from the heart to the brain than neurons leading from the brain to the heart. This indicates to me, as well as to some researchers, that while nature intended a rich transfer of information between the heart and the brain, she believed the heart would have quite a bit more to say to the brain than vice-versa.

The sequence of brain region formation is also of symbolic interest. The most primitive areas develop first, those responsible for instinct and possibly intuition—the reptilian brain and the brainstem. The next area of the brain to form is the emotional brain. The parts of the brain that we think of as giving us "higher functioning" like reasoning, logic, and math ability actually develop last, from the emotional brain. At seven weeks, the embryo is less than one inch long and looks like a tadpole. The heart has been beating for weeks, and the brain is still forming. There is a scaffolding of cells, called radial glial cells, that directs the formation of brain cells from a central zone out toward the peripheral regions of the brain. The brain itself forms from the inside out.

This "hard" science is riddled with symbolism. The heart is the center. The heart is first. The brain, the "thinker," comes afterwards, arising from tissue lying alongside the heart, and is forever linked to it. The instinctual brain is first to develop, and the emotional brain is next. The reasoning brain comes last, out of the emotional brain. The entire development of the brain is a movement from interior to exterior, and interior always remains connected to the exterior.

Nature has priorities. She tells us secrets, hidden in plain sight, about the order upon which the human template functions. The brain is always linked to the heart, and information constantly passes between the two. The heart has much more to say to the brain than the brain has to the heart. If things are going well, the heart speaks and the brain listens and interprets. This is the essence of alignment.

At the opposite end of life, when the heart dies, the person dies. An individual can be "brain dead" and go on living for many years, connected to life force through the beating heart. But when the heart is gone, life is over. A person can be maintained on an artificial heart for only a few hours. Perhaps this is because each person's heart supplies her unique electromagnetic (EM) field. This field of vibration bathes all the cells of our body. Perhaps our individual electromagnetic field provides information about us, as spiritual beings, to our cells and organs. Each human EM field is as distinctive as a fingerprint or retinal pattern. No two are identical.

Mechanical hearts, on the other hand, do not beat in tune with the greater rhythm of life. They are not unique to each individual. Mechanical hearts do not mediate between inner divinity and physical existence. The cells and tissues of the body recognize this. Without a living heart, without their center, they perish. The animating force organizing and linking them to broader, non-physical reality is no more.

Interestingly, further evidence for this notion can be seen in the curious cases of people who have had heart transplants. Transplant patients are frequently emotionally changed from who they were prior to their surgery. Differences in both minor and major aspects of personality have been observed: food preferences, color choices, introversion and extroversion, and language acquisition skill. The transplant recipient becomes a blended being, one in whom the donor heart reverberates in its own unique way in response to the animating force of life.

Our hearts also connect us to one another, and especially to the hearts of others. Scientific studies on touch demonstrate that electromagnetic impulses of your heart affect the brain waves and heart rhythms of people around you.[5] I suspect that the electromagnetic impulses of the heart also provide a path of interconnectivity between humans and all living beings. Animals are often even more sensitive to these field effects than humans.

Why then, in our society, do we give such primacy to the intelligence of the brain while ignoring the intelligence of the heart? The answer is simply this: as we acknowledge the wisdom of the heart and learn to live a heart-directed life, the internal evidence of our spiritual nature becomes overwhelming. Science, until now, has not been willing to acknowledge or address this unity. In diverse spiritual traditions it is the heart, not the brain, that guides the enlightened soul. Those things that fill the heart—joy, passion, awe, and harmony—are the ambrosia that nourishes life force.

The German Christian mystic Rudolf Steiner (1861–1925), founder of the Anthroposophy movement, understood that one of the great transformations of science would come in the twenty-first century as people learned to comprehend the central role of the heart and began to examine life from this heart-centered perspective. Steiner wrote about this almost a hundred years ago, so the time he spoke of is upon us now.

We are ready for heart-centered understanding. We are ready for a new science born of the union of heart, mind, and spirit. These are exciting times, and there is already a lot of great science being done in this arena. One epicenter of this new research in the United States is the Northern California-based Institute of HeartMath.[6] Over the last twenty years, they have examined aspects of the intelligence of the heart and the heart brain. One study looked at the precognition of the heart and brain in more than twenty-three hundred trials. The researchers showed selections from one hundred randomly displayed images to volunteers. Of these hundred images, twenty were negative or upsetting and eighty were neutral. The researchers measured heart-rate activity of the research subjects via EKG (electrocardiogram) and brain-wave activity via EEG (electro-encephalogram) throughout the testing process: before, during, and after the display of each image. Typically, in daily life, when people experience something upsetting their heart rate quickens in response. In this landmark HeartMath Institute study, the researchers were fascinated to observe that participants registered changes in their heart rates several seconds before a randomly generated negative image appeared on the monitors. The random generator had not yet selected the image, but the heart already knew what was coming and responded![7]

This stunning piece of evidence points to a truth that spiritual teachers have been sharing for thousands of years. The heart can guide us, letting us know what is coming and helping us to steer our course in life. As we learn to listen to our heart, we can live life in a more intuitive, more prepared present moment.

For many years I have taught and modeled for patients how to cultivate the relationship between the heart and the mind. I regularly encourage people to listen to their heart when making everyday decisions, including decisions about health and health care choices. The heart can give us important information necessary to run our lives. A life lived in concert with the heart is full of meaning. With the heart fully engaged, the soul's purpose is able to clearly and directly express itself to us.

There are many simple yet profound practices I have cultivated to learn to listen to "the still, small voice" within. The frontier of human expansion lies in this cultivation of a conscious and lively communication between inner and outer being. Contemporary strategies for enhancing the dialogue between heart and mind involve deconstructing culturally derived stereotypes and limiting beliefs. Then we can arrive gently at intuitive wisdom present in the Now moment.

Most great breakthroughs, even in "science," arrive through intuition or flashes of insight. We have all marveled at stories of great clarity that led to transformational discoveries. Tales of "eureka" moments are a consistent theme in scientific exploration, told again and again. These stories always have a common thesis. Epiphanies arrive in stillness, in relaxation, in reverie. The groundwork has been done for the receptivity, the questions have been asked, but the answer does not arrive during striving and grinding. The "aha" comes in peaceful moments.

Friedrich August Kekulé, who discovered the structure of the atom, received a vision of it all at once in a moment of reverie. Robert Louis Stevenson received the entire storyline of his masterwork *Treasure*

Island in a sequential series of dreams. Minister and beekeeper Lorenzo Langstroth revolutionized ten thousand years of beekeeping in his living room one evening in 1851 when he all at once saw "suspended movable frames, kept a suitable distance from each other and a case containing them," and continued remarking, "Seeing by intuition, as it were, the end from the beginning, I could scarcely refrain from shouting out my `Eureka!' in the open streets...."[8] Tesla, Einstein, and most of the greats of modern scientific thought acknowledged that their most sweeping insights came not during plodding and study but at times of relaxation and calm, when, guided by the heart, everything came together.

The science that emanates from awareness of our inner divinity is majestic. Science will flower in the coming era as we embark on exploration of real wisdom rather than continued accumulation of a conglomeration of disjointed "facts." But this new territory requires a science born of love, a science acknowledging spirit. This science recognizes the heart at the heart of the matter, and listens to it. Guided by the heart we create a worldview of wholeness, unity, and love. Love is the beginning and end of everything. It is at the center of our being, suffusing every moment of life. This simple yet radical truth has been observed and shared by mystics and spiritual teachers of every tradition. A new paradigm is emerging; it is the underlying understanding resulting from a maturation of humanity that now is beginning to accept its divinity and interconnectedness. The resulting science, born of love, is and will be so much fun!

TOOLS FOR TRANSFORMATION

1. Since the heart is the metaphorical and spiritual center of our physical existence, you might enjoy doing some exercises to center you in the heart as you read and ponder the ideas in this book. There are many ways to strengthen our connection with divine intelligence.

Your heart sends out electromagnetic waves in all directions, beaming EM energy like the sun beams light. Our individual electromagnetic heart waves can be measured from a distance of about fifteen feet in any direction.[9] One easy technique for centering in the heart is merely to listen to your heartbeat. Sit or lie in relaxation and feel for the quiet rhythm of your heart. You may want to put your hand on your heart or let a few fingers rest on the carotid artery in the front of your neck.

2. Then, while focusing on the beating of your heart, let yourself experience the waves emanating from it. You could enhance this experience by imagining your heart beaming out love, peace, or the best of what you have to offer. You might also play with tracking individual rays like following the twinkling of a star. Remember to just stay in the present—you do not need to judge or analyze this experience while you are engaged in it.

3. Breathing techniques are some of the best tools for centering in the heart. They have been used in spiritual practice throughout human history, with good reason. Breathing techniques assist us in centering our consciousness in the here and now, allowing us to engage in exploration of the life force nourishing us in the present moment. They also help us connect with the rhythms and tides of the physical and spiritual realms.

At any time, but especially when you are agitated, you can visualize your breath flowing to and from your heart. Breathe in to the heart and out from it. Most people find this quite calming. You can also breathe a soothing word such as peace, calm, ease, freedom, or love into and out from your heart. Ease in, ease out, love in, love out, calm in, calm out, etc. Notice how this steadies and slows your heart rhythm when you are anxious, and how this strengthens your feelings of well-being when you are happy.

CHAPTER TWO

Language and Life

THE CONCEPT OF HUMANITY LIVING in harmony with rock and forest, bird and beast, is not new. It is a fundamental and ancient vision that, like the mythological Phoenix, is born anew in each generation. Knowledge of unity resides deep within each of us, nourished by our collective unconscious. It stirs and inspires us. Many stories, legends, spiritual teachings, and artistic images allude to our link with all others. Images and lore such as the dance of life, the great hoop, the eternal wheel, the web of life, and the world tree are found frequently as an undercurrent in art, music, literature, and spirituality. Even the term for the Internet, "world wide web," suggests our interconnectedness at levels beyond the obvious ones.

Often this harmony is described as something lost, a past Eden, a peaceable kingdom, or something we will only find again in some elusive Messianic era. We know that many past civilizations lived in greater harmony with the Earth. Neolithic and hunter-gatherer monuments and artifacts express a seamless wholeness of life, with humans occupying a unique place in relationship with others.

Harmony with the natural world, however, is not lost or mythological, nor is it available only in a nebulous world to come. It is available to any of us at any moment. It is merely our vision that is cloudy, but this is a situation we can correct. We can see the wholeness in any instant, or we can see the lack. Our soul always urges to wholeness.

We have not seen clearly for many reasons. Perhaps we were beguiled by the glamour of the era. Or maybe fear clouded our vision, veiling our true sight. Whatever the reason, we have limited ourselves. We could blame others for this: the media, corporations, politicians, and organized religions are common targets. Perhaps it is true that there are those who prefer us controlled for their own ends. But does it matter? Continuing a cycle of blame just keeps us engaged in the same narrow constraints. It keeps us focused upon "us versus them," in a game where there are "good guys" and "bad guys." We can choose not to play in that game. We can, at any moment, open our eyes, our ears, and our heart and feel the universe of love pouring in.

Despite our small dramas, nature continues its endless cycles of life. All fecundity grows from what came before. It is as if we are dreaming. But at any moment we can awaken to the reality of love. You may ask, how? Language can be one powerful force for awakening or a narcotic droning that dulls our senses. Which do you choose?

Language and Thought

Words are powerful. Words matter. They structure thought as well as what it is possible to think about. They carry significance and create images. Powerful words create an atmosphere and evoke worlds beyond themselves. Although thought is not necessarily ruled by language, functionally we usually think only about things we have language for.

Simple phrases and individual words tell much about a culture. Societies perceive the world differently from one another, and this is reflected in their descriptive language. Many people know, for example, that in the native Eskimo language, Inuit, there are dozens of words for snow. While non-Inuit speakers can describe some types of snow with phrases or sentences, the understanding of snow in the Inuit language is closely related to the Eskimo way of life. Qualities and colors of snow give information about recent and past weather, the migration of animals, and sources of food. Types of snow can be a landmark, a welcome sign, or a warning post. Native Inuit speakers can describe and thus think about snow in ways that speakers of other languages simply do not. An Inuit in conversation with another native Inuit speaker will not muse about the characteristics of the snow she is discussing, she will use it as a descriptor. I, on the other hand, would have to concentrate and apply effort to notice a difference among the various types of snow. I am certain that my observational skills would still fall far short of the facility of any native Inuit child living in a traditional manner.

I recall the power I felt in my youth while studying foreign languages. A native English speaker, I learned Spanish and some French during my middle school and high school years. In college I went to Israel and learned Hebrew as well. As I became more fluent in each of these languages, I realized there were ideas that did not even exist in English, which I could now think about and express. Studying languages opened my mind to new ways of understanding and appreciating the world, showing me the constraints of thinking in just one language. It hinted to me that there are profound thoughts that exist outside language, and I thirsted to know them.

Word Associations

The numerous associations triggered by words are important facets of the significance of language to thought. Individual words weave a web of interconnections that reference external culture and internal psychology. The Rorschach psychological test relies on these types of associations to help researchers understand the individual being tested. Each of us associates words in our own unique way. Our word associations overlap to greater or lesser extent with others in our family, culture, and society, but a snapshot of them reflects a great deal about our individual internal world map.

The connections between words and concepts in various languages also differ widely. That is why it can be notoriously difficult to translate poetry. Even in the best translations much is lost. Poetry is evocative, meaning that part of its purpose is to activate our associative faculty and awaken an epiphany in the reader. Insight gained from poetry is born of the contextual associations of words formed within a matrix of language and culture.

These associations are the reason foreign phrases often pepper our language and idioms flourish. Terms in other tongues convey so much more than a literal translation. A good example is the French term *joie de vivre*. This phrase has now found its way into common English parlance because the French understanding of the term encompasses so much more than just the pleasant words "joy in life." Likewise, the French term *crème brûlée* sounds like a delicious confection while "burnt cream" is far less appetizing.

The associative function of language also underlies the popularity of slang terms. Many concepts do not translate easily because they are only understood fully as a part of the culture that speaks them.

In English we say, if we are working very hard, that we have our "nose to the grindstone" but in Mandarin Chinese one would say, "with liver and brains spilled on the ground." Understanding contemporary idioms explains a lot about a culture and associations within that culture, demonstrating that humans do not all think alike. These and other world-wide idiomatic examples can be found in Jag Bhalla's book *I'm Not Hanging Noodles on Your Ears* (2009). This charming volume gives some wonderful examples of idioms worldwide and helps us take a peek into the cultural nuances conveyed in various languages.

Pure Tone

Language is made up of the meaning of words as well as the sounds of the words themselves. This aspect of language is the pure tones. Sounding of tones shapes thought and consciousness. These precede and shape physical existence. The book of John begins with the famous line, "In the beginning was the Word, and the Word was with God and the Word was God." In life, each day and each moment is a new beginning. In every instant a new world is woven with the threads of vibration, tone, sound, and thought waves.

At the core of each physical thing is vibration. This is illustrated in contemporary physics. All matter vibrates, and all matter has measurable wavelength and amplitude. Consider that even thoughts vibrate. We know the presence of mental activity can be measured in the brain by electro-encephalograms (EEGs). More sophisticated brainwave scanners can show the relative activity in various brain areas in response to specific types of thought and stimuli. A new technology arising from this knowledge has recently been developed by researchers led by Tzyy-Ping Jung at the University of California at San Diego. His team developed a system to interface computers with thoughts, enabling people to dial a cell phone by thought alone.[1]

The power of tone makes more sense when we realize that we *are* vibration. Every cell, every organelle, every atom, and every subatomic particle has a vibrational frequency. Sound, tone, and vibration all create waveforms. Waveforms interact with one another. If they are coherent, they amplify one another. If out of phase, they can cancel out one another.

Because of the underlying vibratory rates and wave patterns, and their interactions, the pure tones and sounds of language are another key aspect of its essential power. Creative application of the evocative qualities of tone has long been the territory of poets, musicians, and mystics. Many mystical traditions exhibit an understanding of the transformative power of the sound of words. Consider the chanting of various tones or mantras in Hinduism, Buddhism, and even Catholicism. In Judaism, the actual sounding of the four-letter name of God is no longer known. Speaking this name was thought to have too much power for ordinary humans. So its true pronunciation was secretly handed down to the religious elite in past eras and is presumed lost today.

In the yogic tradition the power of pure tone is well understood. The sound tone "aaahhh," it is noted, is found in virtually every language as part of the name of the divine being: God, Allah, Buddha, Yahweh, Ahura Mazda (Zoroastrian), Waakan Tanka, Krishna. It is also one of the first sounds a baby makes, and part of the term for "mother" in our early language: ma, mom, madre, emah.

Wayne Dyer discussed the importance of sound meditation for creation and manifestation in his book, *Manifest Your Destiny* (1999). The sound "aaahhh," he explains, connects the third eye, the ajna center of the esoteric body and the area of visionary thought, with the root chakra, which brings all into manifestation. The yogis believe the sound "aaahhh" is the primordial sound of creation; it literally brings thought into physical reality. The sound "ohm," on the other hand, is the sound of appreciation of what has been created.

Cymatics is the study of the effects of sound waves upon physical matter. The word derives from the Greek term *"kyma,"* which means "wave." This emerging scientific field examines the power of tone to create physical structure. All vibration creates. Very high vibrations, it turns out, create forms of great complexity. Sound and tone—in audible and beyond audible range—literally create physical reality and shape consciousness itself.

The German physicist and musician Ernst Chladni did the first cymatics-related experiments in the late eighteenth century. Chladni, who is now considered the father of the field of acoustics, introduced vibration to thinly layered flour and sand on metal plates. He observed the patterns that were formed, finding that low tones (ones slower in vibration) produced simple patterns, while higher tones (faster in vibratory rate) produced increasingly complex patterns. These visual representations of tone were called "Chladni plates."

Hans Jenny, a twentieth-century Swiss physician and naturalist, introduced the contemporary field of cymatics, and the term itself. Jenny began his work with sound images in his youth. As a child he kept pet box turtles and was a keen observer of nature. Jenny was fascinated by the work of Chladni, and he noted similarities between

Chladni plate patterns and common patterns on the backs of his beloved box turtles. Jenny went on to experiment with tones on various media, finding that higher, more complex tones produced a myriad of forms frequently seen in nature and associated with sacred geometry: five- and six-pointed stars, spirals, concentric rings, and hexagonal cells suggestive of honeycomb. Jenny concluded that tone generates the forms of physical matter as well those of consciousness. As if by magic, cymatics bridges the invisible and the visible, concretely demonstrating the vibratory patterns that produce physical matter.

Jenny invented a device to further his investigations, which he called a "tonoscope." The tonoscope allows visualization of the action of sound on physical media. With it, Jenny was able to project onto a screen an image of sounds uttered through a microphone. He published the first volume of *Cymatics: The Study of Wave Phenomena* in 1967. The book, recently republished, is richly documented with photographs of the results of his experiments, which demonstrate the effects of vibration upon various media including liquids, pastes, metal filings, plastics, and powders. A second volume was published in 1972. In an amazing demonstration of the effects of the tonoscope, Jenny showed that a perfectly chanted "Om" creates a series of concentric squares and circles that form the sacred geometric symbol of a yantra.

An exciting application of sound, tone, and cymatic principles is in the area of sound healing. This ancient modality is being reinvestigated and rediscovered with twenty-first-century technological applications. Many spiritual forms of healing include chanting of various restorative tones. Researchers and healers are exploring the science of activating specific tones and wavelengths of light for repair of tissues and restoration of health. Each year there are sound healing conferences that bring together doctors, scientists, musicians, healers, and other visionaries who share the many exciting potential applications of sound in personal wellness, integrative medicine, and transformation of consciousness. As final food for thought, many people believe that the Egyptian pyramids as well as some of the Incan structures were built with the application of a sound technology that is not currently known. The Navajo refer to a time when their ancestral shamans could form sand paintings simply by speaking to the sand. How fascinating to consider that we are heading in that direction once again!

Language and Emotion

Our language conveys volumes about how we feel about things, and it has the capacity to stir our hearts. We have all heard dynamic as well as boring speakers. Consider a captivating speaker. She vividly projects images and paints a scene. There is a gestalt, a wave, a virtual ball of energy that the listener receives and interprets. It sparks other thoughts, images, and sensations. The tone and the words carry us along on our own private journeys, a voyage of discovery based upon our individual inner landscapes.

At times we may not be conscious of the emotional content of our words, or how they relate to our thoughts. The advertising industry capitalizes upon manipulating our emotions to encourage our consumption of products, often playing upon our fears. Buy this product, and smell better or look slimmer, implying a life full of new wonders. This is never overtly stated since that crass of an assertion could certainly backfire. Instead, like a kind of poetry, advertising tries to evoke a mood that feels desirable to the consumer. Buy our pasta sauce and you will feel like you are surrounded by a big, boisterous, loving Italian family. Choose our little blue pill and you will feel youthful and virile as your partner experiences you as affectionate, tender, and sensitive. Not only your sexual function, your whole life will improve.

Written words can carry thought forms and emotional content as profoundly as the spoken word. Think of how a great book can transport you into the lives and landscapes of its characters. A good friend, living in California, recently said to me, "Now that I'm living in Scotland…," referring to a series of novels she was enjoying that are set in Scotland. In a good book, the characters and the scenery are vibrant and alive. We see and perceive them. This is the intention of the writer, and it is a hallmark of good writing.

Poetic metaphor is a perfect example of the wave of thought that coalesces around lively speech. Aristotle taught that poetics ideally evokes emotional catharsis. Public performances of poetic drama served an important role in the cultural cohesiveness of Aristotle's era. Today, the poetry of popular music takes on that role.

Poetics implies a structure, a schema. Within the poetic configuration an emotional world is implied and expressed. The tragic form, Aristotle said, represents men "as better than they are in actual life." Comedy portrays humans as caricatures of their foibles, less than the whole of who they are. As we see people's nobility and grace in the face of difficulties, or laugh at our own self-perceived shortcomings, we have an archetypal experience of self-recognition. Poetry, musical ballads, and drama can evoke feelings of well-being, universal love, and interconnectedness in us, just as they can stimulate feelings of self-hate, loneliness, anger, and isolation. The ancients clearly understood the power of language to shape thought and thus affect expectation, belief, and outcome. They understood the importance of allowing expression of emotion, and thus they used art forms as cultural tools to work psychologically.

Lyrics of the songs we listen to and sing, like the words of poetry we read, do matter—largely because of the emotional resonance that is set up. Think about what you like to read or hear. When you are feeling low, there might be nothing like a bluesy song. When angry, you might gravitate to spiteful music. Happy music, serene music, and songs of love lift our hearts, and we find greater resonance with them when we are joyful or when we seek soothing.

Consider other types of media: How do you feel when you watch the evening news? Read dramatic headlines? Read spiritual literature?

See "human interest" news stories about people rallying to help others? Read stories of animals being inexplicably kind to animals of other species? All words, spoken or printed, can stir our emotions.

Words can be empty as well. Consider a boring book or speaker. In this instance the words are just words. There is no relevant meaning behind them. They fizzle and fade, sounding like blah, blah, blah. The speaker is not seeing any images, not creating any world of wonder for us. We cannot catch the wave, because there is no wave to catch. We are not feeling much of anything.

Boring material has emotional content too, often negative. Given a choice, most people will not continue to read a boring book or listen to a boring speaker. But they will do so, if obligated, or if a feeling of responsibility compels them. They will mouth the words of prayers when they have no heartfelt connection. From a place of fear or duty, divorced from love, some people become complacent and passive, parroting the words and ideas of others.

Layering of Meaning

As we unravel some of what is present in language we find that any interchange involving words contains layer upon layer of meaning and impact. Even a simple discussion between friends can contain many levels of depth. The text is what is literally stated. The subtext is what is meant and how it is interpreted. The underlying emotional assumptions of both individuals, as well as any familial and cultural references sparked, also factor in to any seemingly innocent conversation. So there are many lines to read between, even in an amiable chat amongst friends.

According to Kabbalah, there are four levels of interpretation for any text, indicated by the acronym of *pardes*, or "paradise." This term in both Hebrew and Arabic refers to earthly paradise, the Garden of Eden. *Pardes* reflects the importance of language as a path back to the primordial Garden. The intimation of the term *"pardes"* is that the

Garden is always there, hidden slightly but waiting to be found, available via deeper layers of interpretation.

The term *"pardes"* is also an acronym. The first letter, *Peh*, signifies the word *p'shat* or "simple." It is the storyline as it is presented. *P'shat* is the straightforward text, with no elaboration. A story may sound simple, but any text worth its salt operates on other levels as well.

Dalet, the third letter, refers to *d'rash* and indicates a second, deeper level of understanding of a text: the interpretation. For example, in order to interpret the United States Constitution we require an extensive system of courts, culminating with the Supreme Court. A text might appear straightforward, but interpretations of the meanings and ramifications of that text can vary widely. People's opinions about what a text states can be diametrically opposed. This can be observed in discussion of the spiritual texts of every religion. Religious schisms are usually based on doctrinaire disagreements about the meaning of sacred texts. So there exist many interpretations of spiritual texts such as the Bible, the Koran, the sayings of Lao Tzu, and the *Bhagavad-Gita*.

There are even more possibilities with the letter *Reysh*, the second letter of the word *pardes*, and the third level of understanding. *Reysh* refers to the allegorical level via the word *remez*, which means "hint." There is only a whisper of the *remez* in any text. It is at this level we can open fully to the realm of possibilities and interconnectivities available in a document, or veer off onto our own peculiar tangents. The *remez*, or hint, in a book like *Alice in Wonderland* is alluded to in statements like that of the White Queen: "I've believed in at least six impossible things before breakfast." Is this a hint to readers on how to change reality by changing beliefs, or is it just an amusing line? Or consider the implications of the famous quote of Jesus of Nazareth from the Sermon on the Mount: "If your eye be single, your whole body is filled with light."

The final letter of *pardes*, *samech*, signifies the deepest level of understanding: the *sod*, or "secret." The *sod* is not even hinted at in the text—it is the epiphany that comes or does not come, the eureka! moment that may ensue as meaning unfolds for us. The secret or *sod* level of a text may not even be verbal. It can be a clicking into context of many seemingly unrelated concepts, or a feeling in the heart, or the birth of a sense of knowing. The secret level cannot be taught; its reception is an act of grace and preparation of "the fertile heart." The secret is the most powerful level, yet the most personal, because it changes us from within. There is a sense of knowing born at this level that is unshakable.

Language as a Force for Change

As culture shifts, language changes. As language changes, our thoughts inevitably shift as well. The ability to continue to shift keeps language alive. A language that cannot shift is dead. When Sanskrit became strictly codified by a conservative priesthood in the fourth century BCE and could not be added to or subtracted from, or even pronounced in a newer variety of ways, people stopped speaking it. Not all at once, of course, but over time, as new words, phrases, and meanings were born from new thoughts. The old, strictly codified Sanskrit language became largely ceremonial, and contemporary Hindi dialects were born.

Language must inevitably shift in order to remain contemporary. This changing of language is called "drift." Definitions of words and usage of words drift, as meaning and cultural context shift. That is why English speakers today cannot really understand Old English, other than a few rare terms, even though it was the precursor to modern English spoken from about 500 CE to 1100 CE. As we moved forward from that time and cultural milieu, fewer phrases had meaning for us. Gradually, but eventually, Old English became a foreign tongue. Even the tones and the sounding of Old English letters drifted in the intervening years.

For example, today the poetic words of Shakespeare, penned merely five hundred years ago, require focus, concentration, and interpretation to fully appreciate. In his day, Shakespeare's works were considered intelligent but not difficult; any average person would clearly understand his writing, his allusions, and his tales. To-day the study of Shakespeare has become an erudite endeavor.

We now see huge drifts in language occurring in brief periods of time. Slang gets added to official dictionaries, and old words drop away or their meaning shifts. For example, few people know the meaning of "gloaming," a Middle English word that means twilight, more commonly used one hundred years ago. Most people today think "gay" refers to a sexual preference, though previously it meant "light and happy." Pretty much every American knows which part of the anatomy is the "booty," but few could identify the "hardel" as the back of the hand. (Even my computer's autocorrect no longer recognizes it as a word!)

Language drift, in reflecting cultural changes, has largely been a reactive process. But it can be a proactive process as well. Shakespeare coined hundreds of words for use in his plays including the words eventful, generous, gnarled, monumental, and radiance.[2] He needed new words to convey his ideas and made them up, or reshaped existing words to suit new meaning. We can consciously change language because we choose to do so, understanding the ramifications of our words, the thoughts they convey, and the emotions they trigger.

We can consciously participate in the process of shifting language as individuals, society, and social movements and thereby change our thoughts. In this, we help transform the shape of reality. We change what it is possible to think about, and how we conceive of our world. As we shift language deliberately, we change our own lives and the lives of others. Shakespeare gave us meaningful phrases like "to thine own self be true" and "the milk of human kindness." What metaphors will we bequeath to future generations?

To shift something, it is helpful to notice what is already present, and whether or not it serves our dreams and purposes. Our language evokes powerful emotions. The way we habitually speak of things reveals how we are used to thinking about life. Paying attention to our words, we learn a lot about our underlying beliefs. These beliefs denote how we personally structure reality.

In order to think differently about our health, our bodies, or the natural world, we have the power to use different words, or to change the meaning of the words we already use. We can tell different stories to ourselves about ourselves.

One way to change our thoughts is to consciously change our language. The entire field of Neuro-Linguistic Programming (NLP) is built upon this concept. NLP began in the 1970s as a branch of psychotherapy. Today NLP ideas are popular and widespread in many personal growth arenas like life coaching and the self-help movement, as well as in business and management seminars and political speeches.

The idea of changing language has been applied successfully in industry. The German tycoon Karl Albrecht said, "Change your language and you change your thoughts."[3] He further remarked, "The typical human life seems to be quite unplanned, undirected, unlived, and unsavored. Only those who consciously think about the adventure of living as a matter of making choices among options, which they have found for themselves, ever establish real self-control and live their lives fully."[4] Albrecht came from humble beginnings; his father was a miner and his mother a shopkeeper. Albrecht applied his own philosophy and built a mercantile empire.

Changing language and thoughts to affect life outcomes is a valuable tool for building health. One of the most important perspectives I can offer patients is a glimpse of the correlation between their beliefs about themselves and their health. I encourage patients to take practical steps toward feeling better about themselves, especially in saying nicer and kinder things in their internal conversations. I offer this advice in virtually every patient interaction. What we think about ourselves indicates whether we have the possibility of success. If a patient thinks, "I hate exercise," then he will rarely get off the sofa. This might not be a problem, unless the same person who says, "I hate exercise" also believes that it is not healthy to be sedentary. Their usual internal dialogue could be a self-defeating statement like: "I know sitting around all the time is terrible for my health, but I hate to exercise." Or "I know my addiction to sweets is destroying my health, but I just have no will power." I often work with people to gradually shift self-defeating thoughts to more empowered ones. They turn to statements such as "I am learning to listen to my body and honor its requests regarding nourishment and movement" and "I'm getting better at this and starting to feel better too." I have consistently seen tremendous health benefits resulting from this process.

The Health Care System

It is easy to see how people's self-defeating thoughts, beliefs, and self-talk have negative consequences in individuals. Our unexamined phrases create images for us. The field of psychotherapy is built upon helping people make positive changes in this regard. Our cultural beliefs and expectations about physical health also have profound impact upon the health outcomes we experience.

The language of war is pervasive in Western society, and therefore in Western medicine. This language signifies what is expected and assumed. Warlike images in health and health care indicate a deep mistrust of natural processes, reflecting a perceived lack of harmony between the external world and our physiology. When considering much of the natural world, our tacit cultural expectation is of harm to us, so we must "fight back." Images of war create fear for individual safety, well-being, and one's very survival. Emotionally, fearfulness is deeply disempowering. By engendering fear, modern medicine can undermine patients' confidence, confounding the healing process.

There are many false underlying assumptions in the prevailing "modern" medical system. The term "industrial medicine" is arguably a more accurate description for our current health care machine. These false premises are plentiful and include beliefs such as "we are powerless against disease," "things happen randomly," "there is no meaning in the universe," and "this one life is our 'only shot.'" The modern medical world inculcates limiting beliefs, teaching us to ignore and deny our internal health impulses and to place our faith in "experts." Even public health campaigns are fear-based. In the book *The Individual and the Nature of Mass Events*, Seth (Jane Roberts) astutely remarked that today there is a "barrage of negative suggestions that passes for preventative medicine." We then feel powerless, believing we must try to control the uncontrollable, all the while knowing we cannot possibly do so. So we arrive at the current predicament, where we are afraid of our marvelous bodies.

But we must ask, is this what we want for the healing arts? Do we want to continue to do battle over our physical bodies? Do we want to fear ill health? Do we want to "whip our bodies into shape," or do we want to admire, support, love, and encourage? Do we want to nurture and nourish or compel? Our organs and even our individual cells have wisdom of their own and are able to self-correct and to gravitate toward well-being, if we support them properly.

In popular culture today, there is a tacit agreement that we are at war with many microbes and insects. We rarely if ever see, in popular or medical literature, phrases like "welcoming more bacteria," "enjoying viruses," or "harmony with mosquitoes." When most of us think of bacteria, we think of infections, or "germs" and killing them. Advertising phrases such as "kills germs on contact" seem quite normal to us. When we think of viruses we have images of illness and disease, and when we consider mosquitoes, it is in phrases like "mosquito repellent" and "bug zapper." Few people think of terms like "pollinator" or "friend" when considering mosquitoes.

The Law of Attraction explains that what we focus upon we attract to ourselves. We create our future by the power of our current thoughts. We have become afraid of the microbes, and they have become fearsome. They mirror our current projection. But, under all this, they and we are creatures of love. There is an old saying: "If you always do what you have always done, you'll always get what you've always gotten." I propose we do something different: step out of the war arena and into the realm of cooperation and love.

So What About Peace in Medicine?

While we have gained many valuable things from our current technological era, as we move forward we will need to find the language to describe our inner hopes while allowing and nurturing a new vision. Personally, I want to live in harmony with the natural world. Fighting disease and conquering illness puts us on the battlefield, as does fighting crime and drugs. This is just another manifestation of "battling the infidels." It is war. It's another version of "an eye for an eye leaves the whole world blind." I am bored with the war. Perhaps you are too. Boredom is not a bad place to be. As the teacher Abraham explains, boredom is just one feeling step away from hopeful.[5] They are in the same range of thoughts. And hope leads to lovely thoughts and imaginings. As we indulge more and more in hope, we see more evidence of good things coming our way.

Imagine if we spent our enormous resources and talents creating wonders of beauty, pleasure, and harmony. What if the bacteria, the viruses, and the mosquitoes are all happy cooperative players in whatever game we are playing? Today they have agreed to be villains, because we cast them in the role of villains; tomorrow they are pleased to be friends and collaborators.

In order to think differently about our health, our bodies, and the natural world, we can use different words. We can tell different stories. To make positive changes, we can think and dream about what we *do* want. I recently had a beautiful interaction with a patient I have known for many years. She was describing to me a ceremony done at her church, where each participant wrote down three things they would like to let go of in the coming year. This patient has had many challenges in her life, and she wanted to let go of her health problems, her loneliness, and her financial struggles. As she began to elaborate about each of these, I gently interrupted her and asked, "What would you like to claim in the coming year instead?" It was one of those perfect moments. She realized for herself that focusing on what she wanted to release, retelling the story of her struggle, was in effect not releasing it at all. Focusing on the undesired circumstances re-stimulated the awareness of them and kept them going, continually bringing the past into the present.

Claiming what she really desired, focusing instead upon well-being, community, and abundance, shifted the energy for her. She understood that she could only focus on one thing at a time. Either she was turned toward the solution or turned toward the problem. We were then able to discuss how her financial picture is actually pretty good; she has a loving partner who has been helping her out substantially. Instead of feeling bad about not being self-sufficient, she was able to see that this was the most efficient way that God was able to get the money to her. She realized she had a hand in creating that abundance, and we had similar breakthroughs regarding her health and her friendships. She was able to see that though she has some aches and pains, she is basically healthy and clear-minded at over eighty years young. With this reframing of her circumstances she felt more optimistic about the future, realizing that she could perceive the aches and pains differently to feel better right away, and she could dialogue with them lovingly to discern how they are trying to lead her to greater balance.

Another patient interaction was similar. "Daniel" is a man who is recovering from prostate cancer. He believed that his cancer was related to his fearfulness about masculinity, sexuality, and relationship. In my office, he wanted to talk about more ways of letting go of the fears he believes led to the cancer. I was trying to be helpful, brainstorming with him, but it then occurred to me that our whole discussion was about fear. I pointed out to him that in trying to nudge the fear away he was really drawing it closer, because he kept activating it, mentioning it, and monitoring it.

We never let go of something by focusing on it. Concentrating upon letting go of fear glues us to the fear, precisely because it is the fear we are thinking about, not the well-being. If we feel our cancer is caused by our fear, and we are constantly afraid that we must let it go or we will suffer, then we are keeping our attention on what we are trying to release rather than the improved condition we wish to embrace. By staying focused upon the things we "need to release" we are not releasing them at all. In this circumstance, it is more likely the cancer will recur.

This was a turning point for both the patient and me. The patient stopped talking about his fears and centered himself more fully in the reality he wanted to be living, one in which he felt ease and comfort in his sexual expression. He began to imagine how it might be if he truly felt enjoyment and lightheartedness in his relationships with women.

For my part, I realized that I did not do patients a service by focusing on their worries with them. That amplifies their problems rather than diminishing them. I developed more tools for getting people to talk about what they hope and dream for themselves, and with this metamorphosis, I became a much more effective healer.

TOOLS FOR TRANSFORMATION

Observing language:
1. The practice of observing language is at the heart of this book. Consider your language frequently and non-judgmentally. Notice your words and how they feel to you. Notice your associations and how they feel. Play with words and thoughts emotionally, and steer toward those that feel comfortable, easy, and even delightful.

2. Consider some of the ways culture determines your language and thoughts. Does what you are hearing in the media or from your associates amplify your fear or augment your sense of well-being?

3. Now observe yourself. How many things are you fighting, resisting, or battling in you life? How much do you see your various relationships as a struggle? What are the images you frequently call to mind? How do your images make you feel?

I poignantly remember a Passover Seder at my parents' home just after 9-11. My mom said a long worrying prayer about the perils of terrorism, ending with "I am so afraid." It struck me how she really was afraid, and I was startled to understand that even in the suburbs of Houston, Texas, she felt quite personally vulnerable. I realized that this was how a lot of Americans felt as a result of the news of the 9-11 occurrences—more vulnerable, more fearful, more contracted. I believed it was from watching the news, over and over, and listening to the commentaries, which tacitly encouraged feelings of disempowerment and powerlessness.

I did not feel any of these things. I felt hopeful and optimistic. I felt a great upwelling of love from around the world, and a greater desire to live together in peace emerging from this tragedy. I watch very little news, but I surfed the Web and saw many moving stories of wonderful, caring people working together in a time of great difficulty. Of course, it is fine to follow the news, if that is what you want. But notice how it makes you feel. Notice if you are attracting news stories that make you feel empowered or defeated. Are you feeling how you want to feel? Is this what you want to focus upon? You have a choice, and each choice is meaningful. We are powerful, for we create the world anew in each moment.

What world are we creating by our language, by our thoughts, by our vibrations? What world are you creating for yourself?

4. Take some time to consider these questions now. In the days to come, spend more time observing your language and how it makes you feel. Try shifting what you say, even to yourself, if you notice any feelings of discomfort, fear, or worry. Try to shift to something that feels better. Be creative. Like Shakespeare, boldly coin new words. Watch what happens when these are words of loving-kindness and joy. Jollify and sillify your life. Speak your new delicious words to others. Teach yourself to expect miracles, love, and goodness.

—CHAPTER THREE—

Premises

I STUDIED GENERAL PHILOSOPHY AS AN undergraduate and comparative religious thought in graduate school before shifting gears and deciding upon a career in medicine. After spending many years happily immersed in the nuances of philosophical debate, I realized that all the rhetoric boiled down to one simple understanding: whoever defines the premises wins the argument. The outcome is determined once premises are agreed upon, because shared premises lead to inevitable conclusions. I noticed that many facets of society capitalize upon this understanding. Lawyers, for example, seek to sway the judge or jurors to their set of premises regarding the circumstances of an event.

What are premises? One definition is "a proposition upon which an argument is based or a conclusion is drawn."[1] Another is "a proposition supporting or helping to support a conclusion."[2] A third common definition could be phrased as "something assumed or taken for granted." These definitions demonstrate the association between premises and conclusions, as well as their inherent nature as underlying assumptions. Premises are *not* truths; rather, they are agreements, though at times they are "presumed to be true." The importance of establishing premises for the overall outcome of any discourse is well understood in the branch of philosophy called logic. The *Collins English Dictionary Online* defines logic as "The branch of philosophy concerned with analyzing the patterns of reasoning by which a conclusion is drawn from a set of premises." Once the premises are accepted, any ensuing debate is essentially a formality. It is the establishment of a mutually accepted set of premises that is, in actuality, the real debate.

It is instructive to look at the premises that underlie currently dominant beliefs about reality and see what inevitable outcomes they encode. This is useful both when a person wants to see things differently and when he or she already does see things differently from prevailing beliefs. Our beliefs result from thoughts, and as we have seen in the previous chapter, unexamined thoughts are dictated largely by family and society through the enculturation vehicle of language. We can take a step back and examine our premises dispassionately, allowing them to be seen merely as premises and not as truths. We can ask ourselves questions such as: How do these premises serve me? How do they feel emotionally? Are they comfortable, uncomfortable, or neutral? How does this set of premises mesh with my inner experience of truth? Are these beliefs heart-centered? Do they honor the love that is at the core of me?

As discussed, a central underlying premise of modern medicine is that we are at war. This is not surprising as medicine mimics society at large, where we are currently at war with terrorism, drugs, crime, teen pregnancy, other nations, and poverty, to name just a few targets. In the medical war, the soldiers are medications and medical personnel. The battle is illness and it has many fronts. In medicine there is a constant war with ailments such as heart disease, cancer, and stroke, as well as battles with living beings like "germs" and conditions like obesity and malnutrition. We conquer polio, we battle cancer, we struggle with depression, and we fight AIDS. We use "big guns" to "wipe out" infections and cancers. We are fighting autism, MRSA, and diabetes. We especially fight death. We fight death so hard that one quarter of the funds of our entire medical system are dollars spent upon prolonging life in its last year, forty percent of which is spent in the final month.[3]

A grand premise that underlies our warlike model is the validity of the findings of science. But science is merely a method of inquiry and examination, based upon its own premises. Scientific method is an application of logic. Even the claim of scientific method as a purportedly superior mode of inquiry is itself a premise. Is this really the best way to inquire into the nature of things? Science is not necessarily truth, nor are its findings inevitably true. Scientific facts are only as strong as the premises that underlie them. Often these premises are weak and irrevocably intertwined with the desires and machinations of vested interests.

Consider the numerous studies of cell cultures and lab rats that underlie medical research. Lab rats are a rarified phenomenon, and there are many bizarre strains of them. Some have been bred to grow lots of tumors, usually specific tumors, such as strains of mice that are bred to all have breast cancer. Others have been manipulated to have serious illnesses. None of them could survive in the wild. The experiments themselves are outlandish. Let's take some lab rats and feed this group only one thing for six months. That group we will feed two things. So the group that eats two things does better, lives longer, has fewer illnesses. Does this really prove anything? Does this strike you as uncomfortable, unpleasant, or disturbing? Even when we douse the poor creatures with this drug or that drug, it is not clear to me why we assume we can get any useful information by participating in torturing these Frankenstein products of our own creation. Lab rats and tissue cell lines will show researchers what they expect to see because they have been specifically developed to do just that.

To some, science as it is currently practiced is unassailable. But science is rarely "pure." Most often, scientific findings are manipulated for political and financial reasons. Too often "science" is invoked in the manner that the Bible is invoked by religious fundamentalists. Like the protection of sacredness attributed to any dominant religious canon, no dissent is brooked from the supposedly scientific viewpoint.

But what if science as it is currently practiced, with its deliberate blinders on soul, spirit, and our essential being, is not true at all? What if much of contemporary science looks at reality from a highly limited viewpoint then condescendingly but incorrectly claims that there is nothing more? In a two-dimensional world, movement is only in one plane. Right, left, or transverse, but no up or down. Our current science is similarly constrained. It is a flat Earth, which describes only a small and possibly mostly irrelevant portion of the bigger picture of our infinitely more complex and interesting reality.

We are spiritual beings. Our essential nature as part of a larger non-physical reality underlies and influences our entire physical life. Our existence as spiritual beings is not irrelevant to physical life; it is central to what we are doing here, and by extension it is central to our physical health.

A benchmark scientific tool in medicine is the "double-blind placebo controlled trial." In such a study, supposedly neither the researcher nor the patient knows who is taking a drug or a placebo. This is presumably unbiased and guarantees fairness. Unfortunately, reality is far from this lovely scenario. Even if it were possible to have an objective study, the system of research, especially in the United States, is deeply corrupt. Even when this "double-blind placebo controlled" scenario is followed as well as is possible, generally only results favorable to the vested interests of those who are paying for the study are published. Statistics are then manipulated to represent whatever the financiers of the study want to conclude. Sweeping claims are made for modest findings while large inconsistencies are swept under the rug. A simple Google® Web search for the phrase "science and scandal" returns twenty-eight million results in less than one second.

More importantly, the whole idea of "double-blind placebo controlled" studies relies on a disproved premise that it is possible to have objectivity. A double-blind placebo controlled trial, the holy grail of modern medical research, supposes that it is possible to take the observer out of the field of observation. But the intentions and hopes of the researchers and funders, the method of setting up a study, and the expectations of populations selected to participate will all influence the outcome. We understand from quantum physics that the presence of an observer irrevocably changes and determines what is observed. Objectivity in studies is unobtainable. For example, a recent study published in the journal entitled *Science Translational Medicine* demonstrated that patient expectations and belief in analgesic medications, rather than dosage, determined their level of relief.[4] Building a whole house of cards upon an unstable base is a guarantee that the house will topple. That is what is happening now with the paradigm shift that is underway. I believe some medical studies are potentially valuable, but they are only relevant insofar as they acknowledge underlying subjectivity.

A corollary premise of the medical war is that we are all vulnerable. We are taught to fear our bodies. The underlying assumption is that we have no control over seemingly random and capricious circumstances affecting our health. Yet even scientific studies show this fatalistic view is false. There are many factors responsible for illness, and few or none of them are random. For example, it is widely acknowledged that optimists suffer much less disease than pessimists. One landmark study followed a group of ninety-nine Harvard students for thirty-five years. They were administered a psychological test at the onset, which categorized the students as optimists or pessimists. The study found that the optimists did better in every parameter of life. They had fewer chronic illnesses; they lived longer; had happier, more successful relationships; and were more financially prosperous.[5]

A more recent study, published in a 2008 issue of the journal *Harvard Men's Health Watch*, reviewed a fraction of the many studies that demonstrated the benefits of optimism on health. Findings included these observations: pessimistic men are three times as likely as optimists to develop hypertension and twice as likely to develop heart disease. Optimists undergoing coronary artery bypass surgery had half the complications of pessimists, and optimistic men and women are much less likely to develop high blood pressure.[6]

If we are infinite spiritual beings, it is obvious that illness is meaningful. A better set of questions, with acknowledgment of an underlying spiritual reality, examines the meaning of illness from a broader perspective. This line of inquiry can lead to a more fruitful, health-enhancing dialogue with one's body.

A fear-based model like that of contemporary medicine can lead to undesirable consequences. It thrives upon an us/them dichotomization. It requires "the other," an enemy who is bad or evil and therefore unworthy of respect or consideration. By creating enemies, modern medicine justifies numerous ethically repugnant practices. There is lab testing on live animals. We grow cultures of microbes to see how we can kill them more efficiently. We dump massive amounts of medical waste into the air, water, and earth, blithely ignoring just how long these will persist in the environment, affecting not just other species but also our own future generations. If we examine how we feel about these things, without rationalization, most of us acknowledge that such practices feel bad, uncomfortable, and wrong. We wish for another way.

The premises that we are constantly "at war" and that "we are all vulnerable" are used to justify even more morally abhorrent things. We are told that draconian measures must be observed and civil liberties curtailed. Dubious vaccines can be mandated; children can be forcibly removed from their parents' homes when parents choose "non-conventional" forms of treatment. Environmental health or any mentions of a greater whole, our spiritual nature, or the impact on future generations of current actions are simply shunned as topics of discussion.

The Western industrial medical model justifies its excesses for "the greater good." Yet I must ask rhetorical questions, such as: Is the greater good served when our entire water supply is contaminated with pharmaceutical drug residues? Is the greater good served when virtually every living being on the planet contains Teflon® in their body? Is it the greater good that most mothers' breast milk has enough chemicals and heavy metals to characterize it as toxic waste?

Are the huge stores of radioactive waste from medical imaging and treatments—waste that, by current models, will persist as a blight for hundreds of thousands of years—also just collateral damage of some elusive greater good?

Orwellian in nature, like our societal wars, the medical war provides a never-ending fight. The players appear to change but remain remarkably similar. Because the fear-based thought is perpetually repeated, we get an eternal battlefield. Bubonic plague terrified people of the Middle Ages; smallpox and epidemic flus "wiped out" millions in earlier eras. This year's plague is AIDS, or breast cancer, or prostate cancer, or Ebola virus, or "mad cow disease," or swine flu, or Lyme disease. The means and premises and thus the conclusions of contemporary medical practice are fear-based. There is a disconnection with the Earth and its cycles, and a disconnection from other living beings. We have unwittingly embraced a model of scarcity and fear in our health care system and in our fundamental approach to our bodies.

At its most basic level this means a disconnection with our selves. Contemporary medicine feeds our illusion of detachment from the spiritual beings we really are, and its mechanical model divorces illness from a sense of greater purpose and meaning in our lives. Unsure of any greater reality, we are afraid of death, so we are afraid of living.

Because we get what we expect and we expect a war, disease expands and amplifies from our constant fight against it. Every minor "victory" paves the way for a bigger battle ahead. We are told that we have "won the war" against certain infectious diseases like smallpox, but asthma, ADD, ADHD, inflammatory bowel conditions, cancer, diabetes, autism, and autoimmune diseases have experienced sharp increases in prevalence. So we solemnly fight on, never questioning the basic premises linking health, health care, and war. In the United States, it is estimated that by 2019, on the current track, almost twenty percent of our gross domestic product will be spent on this type of "health care."[7] That means that continuing on this course, one in five dollars spent will go to this absurd battlefield, just as another equally large percentage goes to the equally absurd (in my opinion) battlefield of the military complex.[8]

Many people have observed that, besides being based upon fundamentally flawed assumptions, this current model is completely unsustainable. The U.S. health care system, the most expensive behemoth of its kind in the world, has mediocre outcomes. There are many, many nations spending much less with healthier populations—probably because they have happier populations, but I'm getting ahead of myself!

There is an underlying assumption of scarcity to the currently prevailing social model. It keeps people feeling disempowered, so they are malleable and can be manipulated into being better consumers, more willing warriors, more docile cogs in the workforce. Advertising, even in complementary and alternative medicine, is largely based on promoting thoughts of scarcity, low self-esteem, vulnerability, frailty, and worry.

Medically, we see disease advertised widely in high-budget pharmaceutical ads urging us to consider whether we might "need" the latest snake oil. "Ask your doctor," they exhort, "if *you* might *need* our drug" as if illness were caused by a deficiency of pharmaceutical drugs (or actually prevented by the abundance of them). Because we are afraid and because we feel disempowered, we are sold cures for diseases that later turn out to not even exist, as well as cures that actually cause more disease. For example, it is calculated that in the United States, deaths from commonly used non-steroidal anti-inflammatory drugs have far exceeded the number of deaths from AIDS.[9] Simple, commonplace, over-the-counter medications like aspirin and ibuprofen can damage the heart and gastrointestinal tract. And while they alleviate short-term discomfort, they actually block healing in joints.

There are numerous warning campaigns rife with negative suggestions in the interest of "public health," informing us that all sorts of things can go wrong with us, especially if we are not vigilant. These set up the expectation that ill health and decline are inevitable for most of us. They also set up a lack of trust in our own internal sense of guidance by cajoling us to rely upon various "experts" even if we intuitively disagree with said "experts." The unstated message that we are spoon-fed is "trust others and not yourself."

In the book *The Four Agreements*, author Don Miguel Ruiz calls messages of negative suggestion "poison" and even "black magic." Any media outlet that offers messages that subliminally implant fear, doubt, or insecurity is destructive to our well-being. For real health, we need to ignore the stream of negative suggestion.

The fear-based model is essentially a method of thought control of the many, carried out by the misguided (and self-serving) few. It is actually inconsequential whether this is a deliberate manipulation, as conspiracy theorists would have us believe, or an unfortunate self-perpetuating accident based on enculturation cues encoded by our brains. As we continue to focus on the problem, including musing about the evolution of the problem, we perpetuate its manifestation. It is what we focus upon with worry and fear, or with love and wonder, that really matters. Our energetic offering and how it feels to us is the engine driving all of this. Another view, one taught by diverse spiritual traditions, explains that the reality we create for ourselves is a manifestation of our beliefs.

This discussion is not just abstract. It matters a great deal in terms of each individual's health. Most of us have a lot of premises about our physical body and health that we accept as truth when they are not true at all. Most of us have common beliefs robbing us of the health available to us. We all have stories we tell ourselves about our physical health, based upon these beliefs. These set up expectations. It is as if we are saying to our subconscious mind, this is what I believe; please show me more evidence of these wanted or unwanted things.

Let's take a practical example. Recently I had a little girl in my office who I'll call "Jenny," who had experienced stomach aches for the last few months after a period of high stress surrounding her mother's difficult pregnancy with her little brother. Her mother was now fine and back at home, but she had been hospitalized urgently for pre-eclampsia, a potentially life-threatening complication. I am sure the emotional milieu and stress surrounding her brother's birth played a big part in Jenny's abdominal distress, which developed only two weeks after her mom came home with her healthy baby brother. In the ensuing months the four-year-old child had seen a number of conventional and holistic practitioners who had done multiple stool and urine tests, blood tests, and various alternative tests such as muscle testing. The conventional tests revealed nothing, while the alternative tester diagnosed dairy and wheat allergies by some method that was obscure to both the mom and me. The devoted parents diligently took Jenny off all dairy and wheat for many months and gave her a number of nutritional supplements. However, she did not get better and continued to complain of daily stomach aches. Jenny was not in any day care or pre-school, so there was no chance of that being a stressor, and she appeared to dote upon her little brother.

Jenny stated in my office that "nothing has made this better and nothing will make it better." I found her statement fascinating and significant. Her mom confirmed that she had been saying it for a while. Jenny never had any explanation of why this was so, other than it was her fear. Unfortunately, this small child already had a story, and not a happy one. These types of stories, when they continue, can evolve into actual long-term health problems like digestive disorders. I reviewed all her tests, which showed nothing wrong, and then did a physical exam. While her organs all felt normal, I noticed immediately that she had significant muscular tension, especially in her upper abdomen where she noticed the stomach aches. After the exam, I had a simple but clear understanding of what caused Jenny's discomfort. In the chakra model of the human energy body, the upper abdomen or solar plexus is the area where emotions are integrated. During a period of family crisis, she had taken in a large dose of the fear and worry from which her parents had tried to shield her. She found this emotionally "indigestible" and tensed her abdominal muscles in response. Since she is basically a happy child, the tension just sat in her abdominal muscles, causing discomfort but no real digestive illness.

We did some gentle breathing together to help her relax and notice the difference in how her belly felt before and after. She could see that it felt better and only hurt "a little" after taking relaxing breaths. Jenny and I then discussed the importance of the stories we tell ourselves, and I brought up the idea of telling a different story, one that makes her happier. I asked if she thought it was possible to feel fine in her belly and she replied definitively "yes." When we looked at her whole day, she was able to notice that sometimes she did feel fine, especially when she was busy playing and in the evenings. Together we evolved a story that she could agree with, that her tummy was starting to feel better and soon it would be very happy and she would not even need to think about it. We did not revisit the originally upsetting events in telling the new story. We just moved forward while she learned to relax her muscles through breathing and fun. I also taught her mom a gentle abdominal massage technique that felt very nice to Jenny.

At her follow-up visit six weeks later, Jenny was doing much better. Her tummy only bothered her "a little sometimes" and her mom noticed that it tended to flare when she was emotionally upset about something or did not get her way, or when she was very tired. They were practicing the relaxing breaths together and had made up a silly happy-tummy song that Jenny sang for me. They have postponed pursuing more extensive medical tests at this time since everyone is fairly certain that soon all will be back to normal.

So I ask people all the time to tell different stories about their health, their finances, their employment situation, their romantic life, and their children. This is not to lie to themselves but to tell truly believable and more comfortable stories—stories pointing them in the direction they want to head. While certain factions in science would belittle this as "wish fulfillment," other more expansive scientists have already illustrated the power and efficacy of shifting one's focus to demonstrably improve life and health outcomes. There are many examples. One study that looked at smiling in Berkeley women's yearbook photos found a significant correlation between the display of positive emotions and multiple life parameters thirty years later.[10] Women with broader smiles in their yearbooks were healthier thirty years later! Another study published in the *Archives of Internal Medicine* in 2011 found a thirty percent improvement in survival at fifteen years in seriously ill patients who were optimistic about their recovery at the time of the original illness.[11] Still another study, done at Wayne State University and published in 2010, looked at the smiles of major league baseball players from the 1950s featured on baseball cards. Those with the broadest smiles lived, on average, seven years longer than their non-smiling teammates![12]

Premises are not truth, but since they are generally presented as immutable, those who have not questioned them may accept them as truth. Premises are merely a way for us to organize our thoughts about reality—a handy tool we construct as a platform to build our beliefs upon. Too often, though, we forget that our premises are our tools and begin to confuse them with reality itself. In this case our premises, leading us to defined conclusions, inevitably limit our view of the wider scope of reality.

Premises set up expectations that can manifest in amusing yet poignant ways. I recall a story I heard on the popular public radio show *This American Life* about a young man whose mother always served him chicken for dinner, every single day. He grew up thinking that dinner was chicken and was perfectly content with this situation, knowing no other choice. When he went to college he was amazed to learn that other options existed, that people actually ate a wide variety of foods for dinner, and some of them never ate chicken at all. Eventually he asked his mom why they always ate chicken and she replied merely, "I like chicken." Interestingly, after trying other foods, the student eventually decided that he too prefers chicken, and now it is what he predominantly chooses. So he grew up in an unusual culture where chicken was not only common, it was the only possible outcome. Dinner equaled chicken. Even after learning about and experiencing other "realities"—spaghetti, pizza, curries, steak, omelets, etc.—he remained a chicken dinner eater. Was this inevitable? If he had many different types of dinner as a child would he still strongly prefer chicken? No one knows or can know for certain, but it is likely that he would have developed a broader range of taste preferences.

Once I offered to take my godchildren, aged five and seven at the time, out to dinner. I asked them what they would like. They enthusiastically replied, "Sushi!" I could not have said I wanted sushi for dinner at age five or seven because I never heard of it until my twenties. Still, growing up I had a lot of dinner choices, and fish was often on the menu. So expanding my eating selections to sushi in my twenties was not such a big leap, like it would have been for the young man in the radio program.

Babies are born with enormous potential. Throughout life, some areas of their minds are stimulated and reinforced while others remain undeveloped. Those neuronal areas utilized in each particular child are eventually myelinated. Myelin is a fat-rich sheath that ripens neurons by coating and protecting them. It acts as a biologic electrical insulator. Myelin facilitates and speeds electrical conduction throughout the nervous system.

Myelinated neurons can be seen as a type of superhighway of information transfer that whisks data rapidly through the body. Information is disseminated at lightning speeds as impulses race down myelinated axons then jump to the next neuron via a system of nodal way stations, called nodes of Ranvier. These are hubs for message transfer, like airport hubs, and most of the material relayed at each of them, like a passenger at a busy airport, is just passing through.

Unmyelinated neurons are much more diffuse and slower to excite. They are similar to leisurely local trains with many sequential stops that collect and discharge passengers. But in this case the passengers are packets of information destined for various cells and organs. The information they carry diffuses into body tissues much as train passengers disperse to and from their diverse destinations in their communities.

Myelinated neurons are white in color due to the predominance of fat, mostly saturated fat, in their chemical composition. The white matter of the brain represents a dense concentration of myelinated neurons. The process of myelination in our brain and nervous system happens in several successive developmental waves in a predictable pattern that begins in infancy and continues through our early twenties, possibly longer. After brain neurons are myelinated, they become more or less permanent structures. Brain regions that are not myelinated generally deteriorate at a certain age. The function or potential for function that was present in brain areas that are not myelinated is thought to be lost, although the idea of permanent loss of capacity is itself a premise. Myelinated areas are those that have been stimulated or activated by specific developmental stages. That is why, for example, children who are not exposed to language in the critical first few years, like the famous boy who was raised by wolves, cannot develop it later. There is a huge amount of raw capacity in the developing brain of infants and small children. If no need for a particular faculty or capacity in a child has been observed by the brain or nervous system before a given developmental milestone, then the capacity that was available from that region is not coated with insulating myelin, and the area of raw capacity is literally dissolved away from disuse. It is interesting to consider that we might be able to restimulate the raw capacity if we believed it possible, but are unlikely to find the means to do so while we believe it is permanently lost.

So, in our current understanding, during our brain's early growth and development a set of expectations and responses to the world, based upon what we personally have experienced, gets hardwired into us by myelination. Since each of us has life experience distinct from others, this leads to expectations and interpretations of reality uniquely our own. This is just one way that each of us, quite literally, lives in our own world.

When we are small children we believe that mommy and daddy know everything, and that we are good if we listen to them and bad if we disobey. As we grow older, we individuate, and we usually realize that our parents are merely humans with their own quirks, beliefs, and limitations. Our world expands as we comprehend that they do not know everything. This frees us to draw our own conclusions. With expanding consciousness, like children growing beyond their parents' narrow beliefs, we inevitably see the limitations of many of the premises we assume, and we grow beyond them. That too is the nature of the human experience and may be hardwired in our brains as well, in the construction of the right and left hemispheres and other structures.

I describe all this not to veer from the topic of premises into the nature versus nurture debate. I believe that ultimately, as spiritual beings manifesting in a physical reality, we can and do transcend all of it: culture, social structure, and the predispositions of our genetic heritage. Even our myelination patterns, I believe, will be found to be more malleable than was previously thought. These are prominent forces shaping our experience of reality, but there is no known basis for a premise of determinism in any of these factors. There are, for example, documented cases of individuals with a type of hydrocephalus, a disorder that fills the brain with fluid, who have only a thin rim of brain tissue but display normal intelligence.[13] Genetic, biologic, and cultural determinism are just another set of premises that lead us into a fearful and worried state of acquiescence to the status quo.

So how do we choose new premises? In my medical practice I find that each patient must develop the confidence to make these choices for themselves. I frequently explain that old premises are not bad. They are just old. They are like the winter coat you had when you were six years old. At that time it fit comfortably and was snuggly and warm. But if you tried to fit into it as an adult, it would be too confining and quite uncomfortable. Some of our old premises about our world and ourselves are similarly constraining. They were useful in their day; in fact, often they were the very best choice at the time we adopted them. But when they begin to feel tight and binding it is time to let them go.

My process has mostly been an internal one, informed by voracious reading. My individual path has included mystical contemplation, personal paranormal experience, study of leading-edge modern physics, and study with various teachers. All led me back to the same understanding about premises that began this chapter. We access reality only through consciousness. Many others have observed permutations of this. In 1944, quantum physicist Max Planck presciently observed a similar phenomenon. He stated:

> As a man who has devoted his whole life to the most clear-headed science, to the study of matter, I can tell you as a result of my research about atoms this much: There is no matter as such. All matter originates and exists only by virtue of a force that brings the particle of an atom to vibration and holds this most minute solar system of the atom together. We must assume behind this force the existence of a conscious and intelligent mind. This mind is the matrix of all matter.[14]

As a mystic, I have directly experienced a basic premise of our reality quite different from the prevailing model of fear and scarcity. I see that love is the fabric from which every contrasting thing is woven. This knowledge is available to any of us any time we are willing to wake from the nightmarish dream of our limiting beliefs.

Reality is what we make it. There are many worlds, many lives overlapping on this planet, and each of us floats around in our own bubble of creation based upon what we observe and what premises form the conclusions we draw from our observations. Our premises determine our attitudes and beliefs about what we are doing, and what aspects of life experience we will focus upon next. We create our next experiences from the direction and focus of our previous thoughts and emotions. We each create in our life experience what we believe to be true. In groups like families, communities, and cultures much of this content becomes coherent and appears similar, but it is never identical, even in twins raised in the same family. By our fresh experiences, both the positive-seeming ones as well as the negative-seeming ones, we learn what it is we do or do not want in future events. Thus we grow, and thus we shape reality, as individuals and societies.

We create ourselves and the whole of our life experience. The mind is the matrix of physical reality. Our physical reality is one enormous "lab" for trying out creation of various thoughts and beliefs. We experience the energetic flavor of whatever we, as individuals and cultures, feel and focus upon long enough. If we believe life is tough, we will have ample opportunities to play that out, learning just how rough and unfair life can be. If we believe health inevitably declines with age, then we expect frailty and disease. But if we expect that life is a joyous self-expression, if we understand we have more control and freedom than we have ever previously allowed ourselves, then we can live flourishing expansive lives that might seem truly miraculous to others who do not yet have the same understanding. Essentially, then, *we* create the premises, or inherit them from our family and culture, and follow them to their logical conclusions, where we observe the outcomes as the content of our life stream.

We have long forgotten that there are premises that forge our lives, and we control and select them. Thus we may seem to be stuck in loops of undesirable and even terrifying outcomes. Many people simply do not believe we have any power over "external circumstances." This misunderstanding can eventually lead to hopelessness or despair, or to desperate attempts to control events and other people in order to make us more comfortable.

As a healer, I look at this conundrum daily. Most patients do not have a clue about how they might be creating their experience. Most have never heard or thought about the whole question. To most, poor health does seem to be caused by chance, bad genes, bad luck, environmental factors, virulent "germs," or poor dietary or lifestyle choices. They believe that disease is externally generated. There are many "experts" out there, even in complementary and alternative medicine, who happily reinforce the premise that things just happen to us, or happen to us for various reasons unrelated to one's subjective reality, internal sense of the world, or underlying beliefs and expectations. Each of these experts has their own take on what is happening and what is the cause. So, it is explained, you are ill because you ate this food or did not eat that one, or because you smoke, or because you were exposed to this toxin, or that bacteria.

Because we have accepted the premise as a culture, it is acceptable to believe that the locus of control of one's health is outside one's individual consciousness. We believe that germs, disease, heavy metals, mutation, radiation, corporations, poverty, malnutrition, or "bad" genes have caused an undesirable thing to happen to us.

Most patients cannot fathom that they are running the show. They certainly do not consciously desire the health problems they are experiencing. Suggesting that their thoughts and focus directly affect their health outcomes or other life experiences can be interpreted as "blaming the victim." For many people, this perspective is implausible and may even seem cruel. The thought of changing their beliefs and premises just adds to the overwhelm of their serious health problems.

Some patients are not ready for or interested in this message. That is okay. Everyone is on their own journey and the pace, the tempo, and the details belong to them. The journey of each of us is meaningful and unique, and it is not my job to dictate to anyone else the direction they travel. I know we are spiritual beings living a physical existence; I know illness is not a punishment but rather a communication of a misunderstanding. I also know it is not my job to persuade others of what I believe. My understanding is for myself and for others who desire that perspective. My job as a physician is to bring ease, not to create more stress.

So I try to soothe these people, and encourage you to do the same for those you know who are not open to or ready for this message. If someone has not asked a question, he or she is certainly not interested in the answer. If the concepts in this book resonate with you, that is wonderful! You are on an amazing and fun journey, and the rest of this book can help you and spark excitement about a world we can create together. Being skeptical or disbelieving is fine too. We are eternal beings. At some level there is just One of us. We are all connected, and everyone, every part, will eventually be soothed. Do what you can to feel better now. Feel more aligned with your heart now. Live your life more authentically as the highest and best you. Perhaps you can try to gently, softly soothe the dis-ease, the lack of ease, in others you know and care about. Simply feeling happier, in any moment, is its own reward.

There are lots of signs that a growing number of people are aware of the central importance of thought, focus, consciousness, and vibration. I have resonated with the teachings of Abraham-Hicks for many years and am pleased to observe the growing popularity of concepts such as the "law of attraction" and "creating one's own reality." These ideas are becoming much more mainstream, popularized by films like *The Secret* and *What the Bleep Do We Know?*, books like *How We Choose to Be Happy*, and courses such as "Awakening Joy" and "Manifesting the Reality You Desire."

Even Oprah devoted significant airtime to delicately dancing around this topic. She has hosted an online course with Eckhart Tolle, interviewed Esther and Jerry Hicks on her XM radio show, and featured Louise Hay and teachers from the movie *The Secret* on her TV show. It is apparent to many of us from diverse fields that we are undergoing a paradigmatic shift, one in which we acknowledge our own power as creators. Our premises are changing, and so the world, malleable only to thought, is changing too. This is a grand opportunity for us to reconsider the whole of what it means to be human, along with the meaning of health and disease.

Medicine and healing are undergoing a change as well, though you might not know this from the conventional medical "business as usual" model. To reiterate, the fundamental premises of the prevailing medical mode are based on an old paradigm describing illness but not health. We have developed brilliant technology to fight a war existing only in our minds. Yet the fear and war-based train of thought, whether in society or in medicine, is a path leading to nowhere we want to go. But this is not another book explaining how bad it is. When observing things we do not like, consider their positive promise. This gives us information about what we really do want.

I propose a vision of an alternate view that is in the process of being born. This view is one of harmony with our natural world. It combines a loving knowledge of biological systems with ease and connection to our inner and outer environments. This is a view that genuinely feels good, maybe even better than good. It feels like grace, like magic, like wonder, like love. Borrowing the words from the story "Goldilocks and the Three Bears," it feels "just right."

How do we get to this new vision? Thinking about problems currently inherent in the world can feel overwhelming. Lacking an alternative approach, initially we opt out of thinking about it at all. Not focusing on the problem is actually quite a good starting point for changing one's focus, because you move away from the stream of worried focus that amplifies the undesired situations.

But we do have so much untapped power. As Margaret Mead eloquently stated, "Never doubt a small group of thoughtful people could change the world. Indeed, it's the only thing that ever has." Consider that this small group of people includes you and me. Consider feeling empowered to dream a new world into being. Small groups expand into larger groups. Whole movements grow from individuals sharing dreams of something better, and knowing a path will open for them. We can consciously drift thought patterns, just as we can consciously drift language.

Imagine what feels good and feel the goodness in it. Imagine a health care system in harmony with the natural world, where there are many desirable choices. There is no need to know the details of how this will look. Just begin in the wisdom of your heart. This new medical system, this society based on harmony and respect, is an evolving vision. It is clear, though, that the greater good, as a bottom line, must feel comfortable. It does not leave us uneasy, with thorny ethical questions looming. We recognize good by our emotional feelings of well-being.

Native American cultures (specifically, the Iroquois confederacy) considered the effects of their current actions upon the next seven generations. The current industrial model often forgets to take into account (or conveniently disregards) the next seven *years*. Short fiscal cycles have long consequences. A "greater good" that feels bad is a lie. This false promise of good brings much destruction in its wake. True good is not seemingly good for some and terribly bad for others. It serves the whole and factors in unconditional love; it is good for all, including the future generations of both the prince and the peasant.

The strength of philosophy is that it allows us to model the workings of reality. By applying different premises we observe different outcomes. So, in doubting the premises of industrial/corporate "modern" medicine, I propose different ones that fit more with my understanding of underlying reality. These spiritual-sounding premises actually gel better with the perceptions of leading-edge quantum physics than do the premises of the current (but antiquated) paradigm. My premises also fit reassuringly with the wisdom offered by traditional societies that managed to flourish in balance with the Earth for countless thousands of years. The first of these new premises is the understanding that we are spirit beings, non-physical energy, having a physical existence. The French Jesuit mystic Pierre Teilhard de Chardin said, "We are not human beings having a spiritual experience. We are spiritual beings having a human experience."[15] This saying is practically a bumper sticker here in Northern California where I live, but I think the implications of this well-phrased insight are taking on new meaning in this era of exciting change and growth. If we are spiritual beings having a physical existence, we have a whole new ball game. Then our lives are about who we really are, spiritual beings, and our physical life is meaningful in what it offers to our total self. We grow by bringing more of this total self into the discourse of everyday life.

We are spiritual beings in physical existence, and while we know ourselves as physically alive and perhaps feel that we are finite, there is a greater, broader part of each person and perhaps each creature and plant that is eternal. As eternal divine beings, we are infinite. We cannot ultimately be harmed. We cannot really die, though we do eventually cease to live physically on this Earth in our current form. Our purpose in living a physical life is the soul's purpose: joy, expansion, and the creation of greater love. The Dalai Lama simply and eloquently stated it thus: "The purpose of our lives is to be happy."

Some other "new" premises I would like to propose follow from this first one. They help us revisit our relationship with the natural world and re-envision our health care system. The second premise is "The Universe is intelligent." This is the position of the Bioneers, a wonderful organization devoted to exploring new ecological and holistic solutions to environmental and social issues. Their mission statement is as follows: "*Bioneers* is inspiring a shift to live on Earth in ways that honor the web of life, each other and future generations." Their website used to pop up with these words (paraphrased): "it's all alive, it's all intelligent."

So a corollary to the second premise is "Everything has consciousness." Not just living things, but every atom and every molecule. We can interact with this consciousness. This ancient understanding perhaps enabled our ancestors to build the great pyramids with sound, a feat that today seems miraculous or impossible. There is potential for our future generations to enact similar wonders.

From this understanding, there are so many exciting possibilities. If there is an underlying intelligence with which we can interact, then the nature of our discourse with nature is inevitably changed. In the next chapter, I share with you one of my personal experiences involving communication with ants, and its world-changing implications for me.

A third premise, found in many sacred texts, is one I discovered in my own journeys: Divine Love is the basis of reality and the fabric of creation. Most people in the world belong to one religious group or another. This teaching is at the core of almost all of them, yet few people understand its vast implications. Every thing and every one is Love, from a tiny microbe to the people of a neighboring or distant country. Everything you see, everything and everyone you interact with, is part of this Divine Love.

A fourth premise is the "Law of Attraction." The now-familiar term "law of attraction," made popular and mainstream by the teachers Abraham-Hicks, states that we live in an attraction-based universe.

Everything is drawn to that which is vibrationally like itself. I questioned this idea when I first encountered it. What about magnetism, for example? North and south attract one another while north and north are mutually repellant. What about the old saying "opposites attract"?

I was slowly convinced of the reality of the Law of Attraction, through years of observing my own experience as well as the experience of those around me, including my patients. I saw the world conform to my expectations and beliefs in small and large ways. The underlying key here is vibration and how things match on an energetic or vibrational level. North and south do match, vibrationally, like lock and key or hand and glove. They are of the same energy; both are aspects of magnetism, ultimately of the same purpose, like two sides of a see-saw.

In philosophy, corollaries are what follow premises. If we believe "if A then B," and we accept "if B then C," then we deduce "if A then C." From the premises of "everything has consciousness" and "law of attraction" comes the corollary that the universe continuously mirrors, through the manifestation of our life experience, exactly what we are projecting or "vibrating." This is so whether the manifestation is desired or undesired. Like attracts like. Experiences that concretely demonstrate our predominant thought and belief patterns show up in our life stream. If we think mostly thoughts of harmony and well-being, we thrive. If we dwell upon thoughts of self-deprecation or scarcity, we suffer. Well-being is always an option as we become able and willing to shift.

So disease is just dis-ease. In illness, there certainly is a lack of ease. Dis-ease means we, as individuals or societies, are not in harmonious balance within ourselves. We are not feeling the ease that our essential nature is always offering to us. Ideally we notice our lack of ease in emotional feelings of discomfort. But generally we override our subtle levels of awareness of discomfort for a myriad of supposedly good reasons. It is apparent in adults that illness relates to our thoughts, beliefs, and behavior because it is usually from these thoughts and subsequent emotions that ease or the lack of it develops.

In a medical practice lack of ease is not hard to find, if we ask the right questions. In my office I listen to patients with a myriad of health problems. Often they complain about unfulfilling work, unhappy personal relationships, or low self-esteem. Frequently, the more hopeless and disempowered they feel, and the bigger the unrealized dreams and hopes, the more dire the illness.

When we ask different questions, we get different answers. When we, as individuals, communities, or cultures, are not attending to ourselves and to our divine inner being, we are not being true to ourselves, and illness may develop as a clarion call reminding us of who we really are, what we planned for our individual life, and what collectively we plan for human civilization.

Lack of ease extends to the paradigms offered by our culture. As we have seen, the prevailing cultural milieu is often fear-based, and yet, I believe, in the recesses of our hearts we know ourselves to be love. The fact that we are not at ease, not nearly, is clearly reflected in the predominant health conditions of our society. This is not blameful. In fact, we are always evolving, always expanding, so our soul, our inner being, is always slightly ahead of the physical self, calling us forward into our expansion. When the gulf between who we are as expanded spiritual beings and who we are as physical beings grows too wide, disease manifests.

I do not, however, pretend to have a pat response to profound questions of why this individual or that community experiences exigencies in its life in a particular way. There are health conditions, such as congenital diseases and illness in small children, which seem difficult to accept or understand. Among many possibilities, such illnesses may be consciousness physically mirroring to us our collective societal and cultural discomfort. I address more of my thoughts and speculation about these profound questions in Chapter Ten, though I certainly do not have all the answers. I merely understand that my worried or angry musing about such problems gives me no respite. In my physical form, I am not consciously inside the growth processes of others. I do not stand in the place of their soul and make their decisions about their path and their subsequent expansion. So I cannot claim, from my limited human perspective, to have an answer to the meaning of each experience as it filters into individualized personal reality. I do know that from a place of oneness, all is well, and we are eternal beings, expanding into ever greater love. It is that space, at the heart of us, which sustains and nourishes each of us despite our apparent separateness.

A final corollary is: If love underlies all levels of reality, and if everything contains a measure of consciousness, then the natural world holds no malice toward us. Malice is not possible because every physical thing is made of the fabric of love. The natural world is part of all that is, and all that is, is made of love. Therefore it is not even possible that the natural world is simply neutral toward us. We are all in a dance of consciousness, of unity in infinite diversity, of loving co-creation. We exist as part of a cooperative community of life imbued with the essence of the divine. Love, the essence of the divine, suffuses all things.

If we accept these premises, then we must conclude that there is a place for all things. The natural rhythms we observe are correct. Death as well as birth is sacred. So there must be a value to spirochetes and viruses and creatures like rats and roaches that we have previously characterized as "vermin." They are not "the other," bad, dangerous, or wrong. We were not born to live in enmity with the natural world. Bacteria, fungi, spirochetes, parasites, viruses are all as much a part of the natural world as kittens, roses, honeybees, and oak trees. The world is a place of love, not a place that wants to harm us.

We have been barking up the wrong tree for a long time. Nature keeps beckoning to us, respectfully requesting, "Pay attention, and look at me!" We will not find our way through a science of hate and fragmentation. We will not find peace on our planet while we continue to subdue, dominate, or conquer. We can develop a science of love, a science of wholeness. Children know this. That is why they love magic. Magic is real, as real as we knew in our youthful hearts. The world is alive. It breathes with me and within me.

Based upon these new premises, I propose a model of peace in the realm of medicine. If we understand that we are infinite beings who cannot really be harmed, then the terms of our dialogue with our physical body are radically altered. Illness is a manifestation of imbalance with our self, with our inner purpose, or even possibly a mirror of a larger social imbalance. Illness is meaningful in the life of the soul. Illness is not to be feared, it is not a punishment for misbehavior. Instead, it is a concerted effort of our bodily cells in cooperation with the natural world to remind us as individuals and societies of who we really are. Illness calls us home to our true self, reminding us to attend to the connections among our soul, our society, and our physical human expression. Illness gives us a nudge, as gently as we are able to hear it, toward profoundly greater health.

Admittedly, this does not always feel gentle, because many of us have gotten out of the habit of listening to our inner voice. We make the illness the problem and a further object of fear. The illness becomes more evidence of our lack of control. The magic key to healing is to find inner peace, or to steadily move toward it. We have the power to change what really matters: our thoughts and beliefs. We are the only ones who can shift our own perspective.

Make peace with illness, as best you can, because the illness is not the enemy. In fact, there is no enemy. There is only ever-evolving consciousness and ever-expanding love. The key is in letting go, looking in the mirror and beginning to see how radiant you are. Let yourself express more of the love that you are. To heal, you may have to give up your pet gripes and dissatisfactions. You may have to stop complaining or revise strong judgments you hold. You may have to let go of believing and reminding yourself that you are not good enough. Consider that you may be whole and fine just as you are.

True healing is an inner journey, not an external one. While you are in the process of becoming greater love, allow yourself to use tools that are available to find relief. Medications and remedies as well as breathing techniques and visualizations can help. Relief is important since it is usually easier to focus on our true nature, or focus upon our well-being, when we are not suffering from a pounding headache or hosting a large tumor. But we do ourselves a disservice by confusing the tools with the transformation. We can wake up. We are waking up. These are new premises that empower and honor our true freedom and creativity. These so-called new premises are not really new at all, for they are part of the eternal flowering of love available to us at all times. They are timeless, and the time for them is **now.**

TOOLS FOR TRANSFORMATION

1. Question your assumptions. I often ask patients questions such as "What makes you happy?" "What do you think happens to you after you die?" "Are you more of an optimist or a pessimist?" and "Do you believe things generally work out for you? Or do you feel life is a struggle?"

2. List your assumptions as you discover them. Get a journal and write them down. Notice emotionally which ones feel best. If possible, replace the uncomfortable ones with different, more harmonious beliefs.

   Consider trying this test: Breathe into your heart as described in the first chapter. Then try to feel the assumption there. Does it give you warm, cozy feelings? If it feels good in your heart, it is good for your health. If not, reconsider your assumption.

3. For an entire day, notice and list the many things you assume. At the end of the day, evaluate whether or not you want to keep them. For example, on a given day you may assume things about others and yourself such as: "she doesn't like me," or "he thinks I am stupid," or "I'm such a loser," or "she thinks I am talented," or "he seems like a kind person." Write them down, whether positive or negative. You can decide later if you like those assumptions based upon whether they feel comfortable. Of the ones you dislike, what would you prefer to be the case? Of the ones you like, what is pleasing about them?

4. Find ways to soothe yourself, especially if you are working with a frightening or life-threatening health situation. Try some of the breathing exercises. See if you can connect with your heart. Remember, illness is not a punishment. You are not bad, but you are not a victim either. You are divine intelligence, manifesting as a physical being for joy and for love. You are eternal. No real harm can come to you, even if you die. Your body is speaking to you as a vehicle of your soul, of who you really are without the veil of illusion. Your body is communicating in the gentlest way you will hear or notice. It is inviting you back into harmony—even though, from your current perspective, this may not feel gentle at all.

There are numerous potential roads leading to harmony. Medications and surgery may be part of your road and that is fine, bless them, but they are tools not the cure. The cure, the magic, is you: your alignment with you. Eventually we all come into this alignment, though for some it is finally achieved in the process of dying. That is all okay. You are Love and deep inside yourself you know this.

—CHAPTER FOUR—

Respect

IN NORTHERN CALIFORNIA, WHERE I live, ants come indoors during the cold rainy winter. They take up residence in houseplants, congregate around the kitchen sink, swarm the trash can, and partake of the pet food. My partner and I used to be like many Americans, blithely killing ants because they were in "our" home. Neither of us had previously lived in an area where the ants moved indoors each year, and we felt affronted by their persistence. I perceived this as an "invasion" and took it personally, even though I sensed this was an unhelpful perspective.

In our first years in California we tried "environmentally friendly" ant-repelling chalk from China, which, it turns out, was not actually environmentally safe at all. We also sprayed the ants with a natural oil that killed them on contact and was supposedly safe for "us" and our pets, and we also just squished thousands of them. The oil blend was the most effective but I hated the smell of it. The nauseating odor would linger for days. I felt frustrated, but I never questioned the "need" to kill the ants. We achieved a little success in protecting the pet food by putting moats of water around our pet's bowls. The physical barrier prevented the ants from overrunning the pet food.

Then, several years ago, Star and I realized that neither of us felt good about killing the ants. Several things had happened in the intervening years. We had become avid students of the teachings of Abraham-Hicks and began to pay a lot more attention to how we felt. We began to notice that the war with the ants felt quite bad. We also had read Joanne Elizabeth Lauck's beautiful work *The Voice of the Infinite in the Small*, as well as Machaelle Wright's *Behaving as if the God in All Life Mattered* and were profoundly moved by both. I attended many seminars at the Monroe Institute and had deepened my daily meditation practice.

In noticing our feelings, respecting the life of the ants felt much better than killing them. And from our resultant expanded perspectives, we began to think instead about what was good about ants, and to look for nicer aspects of the current situation. We noticed that we were doing our dishes as soon as they were dirty. We were definitely keeping the kitchen cleaner. This was pleasant because it is always nice to come into a sparkling clean kitchen. We also began appreciating things about the ants themselves. Ants are very industrious, helpful to one another and great cooperators. I decided that dialoguing with the ants was a better alternative than the previous program.

My initial attempt at communication was a unilateral directive, and I still missed the point. I requested that they stay outdoors and promised I would leave them alone there. I felt no animosity toward them, or maybe I really still did somewhat, but I wasn't going to kill them. I had declared a unilateral truce. This felt a lot better. With that improvement in my comfort level, I tried to negotiate by listing my demands. "I will not kill you, but I want you to leave the house." "Please do not disturb the trash can."

This did not seem to have an appreciable effect on them. As Star pointed out, there was no real dialogue. I had talked *at* them, just expressing my own viewpoint. My only bargaining chip was that I would not kill them, but this was no real offer. This, for me, had uncomfortable parallels to much of the United States foreign policy. "We could kill you or take over your government, but we will not, for now. Do what we say, though, or perhaps we will reconsider." Anyway, the ants responded to my vibration and they understood, in whatever way they do, that mass killing had moved out of the realm of possibility for me, so I was not really threatening them either. I was just saying what I wanted, and since they do not actually understand words, this probably sounded like the energetic version of whining.

I then resorted to cajoling. "If you leave the house, I will put food outside for you every day. I will give you the pet food you like so much." Still there was no noticeable difference. I put dog kibble out-side which the ants ate outside, but they hung out in the house, too. I tried sealing all the places I thought they might be entering with a brightly colored paint. I had not essentially changed my position; I wanted them to live outside. Although offering something, a food bribe, I was really continuing to make demands.

But then something else began happening as well. I became fas-cinated by the ants and curious about their ways. Why do they have this trail and not that? Why do they, who are usually so industrious, sometimes gather tightly in a circle, close together on the counter top, so they form an almost solid mass of ants, and just remain there unmoving? Why do they choose to live in some plants but not others? Why are there a few ants that are so much bigger than the other ones?

I noticed that they helped their fellows. If an ant was injured, oth-er ants would come and try to heal it. If an ant died or was killed, they carried the body back to wherever they went. I saw how strong they are, carrying grains of food almost as large as their bodies, or carry-ing another whole ant. I began to love their cooperation and society. I got a big magnifying glass and would watch them through it for entertainment. Not disturbing them, just observing and appreciating. Somewhere in there, I stopped trying to get them to move outside. I recognized that it was cold outside, and raining for days on end, and understood it was reasonable for them to want to be warm and dry. Plus, I now liked them; they were kind of like fascinating miniature pets. Then some odd things began to happen. They "spontaneous-ly" stopped swarming over the pet's food and restricted themselves mostly to the compost bucket. I hadn't asked them for anything, but of all the places they could be in the kitchen, I did feel perfectly fine about them being in the compost bucket.

If they were in the sink and Star or I planned to wash dishes, we'd let them know what was going on, saying, "I'm going to wash the dishes in about an hour, so if you do not want to be washed down the drain, you might move out of the sink." This was without anger; it was with respect and love. We actually wanted them to move out of the sink, because we needed to wash the dishes but did not want to harm them.

An hour later, ninety percent of them had left the sink. This happened over and over again. When a housekeeper was coming we started to explain to the ants a day in advance, "Someone will be here tomorrow and will wipe up the counter top next to the compost bucket, so it is probably not a safe place for you." Then I started to hear them respond, in my heart. "Where would be better?" they asked. I thought about it and mentally replied, "The bathroom windowsill would be fine, and no one will disturb you there." The next morning I awoke to find only a few ants in the kitchen, and loads of them on the bathroom windowsill.

Later that day, after our housekeeper left, the bulk of the ants returned to their kitchen trails and the compost bin. I felt a mix of emotions, all positive—amazement, peace, and love. The world had changed profoundly.

I told this story at an Abraham workshop some time later. I was not exactly sure why I felt prompted to tell it. The format at these workshops is that people raise their hands if they have a question; and if they are a "vibrational match," meaning they are aligned enough to be noticed by Abraham, they may get called on to ask their question in front of the crowd. In these workshops there might be three hundred to seven hundred participants, and at any given opportunity, a hundred people are raising their hands with a question. In the course of an average day-long seminar, only about ten or twelve of these are called on to come and ask their questions in the "hot seat."

Everyone learns from each question, and from how Abraham meets people energetically and responds. When I arrived at the workshop, I did not have any burning questions. I love the workshops, love to see how Abraham sees people and loves them, helping them to see their own light and move their energy to a better place. I like going into the "hot seat" because I always feel like I am getting a vibrational fine-tuning sitting there. You get a lot of that just being in the workshop, but for me, the hot seat is like an intense beam of positive energy.

So, I had internally stated an intention to know when and if it would be a good time for me to be in the hot seat, and to feel inspired to raise my hand if appropriate. Various questions flickered through my mind throughout the day and were answered in the responses given to other questioners. I did not raise my hand. Then I began to think of the ants. I had already figured out so much of this, and felt the wonder and the love in it all. I was, in fact, well into writing this book. Then my mind began to formulate a question that involved telling an abbreviated version of this story. Then I knew, clearly and confidently, that I would be called upon next, and of course I was.

I was one of the last questioners of the day. Many people came up to me afterward and thanked me. Some shared stories. One man, for example, told of how he had struggled with slugs in his garden. He killed them lots of ways, putting down traps, using iron, and just squashing them. Then he read Machaelle Wright's book and asked his garden, "What should I do?" He heard, in his heart, "First, stop killing the slugs." He said, humorously, that he knew this wasn't his own voice because at that time he enjoyed killing slugs. Still, he stopped.

He planted twelve lettuce plants. The slugs ate two of them completely, down to the core. They did not touch the other ten. This pattern has continued now for seven years. Eventually he was in his garden one day and wondered what the *deva*, or spirit, of his garden looked like. At that moment, a hummingbird flew up to him, inches from his face, and hovered there. Since then, when he speaks to his garden, he addresses the mental image of the hummingbird.

One day he was thinking about the garden and asked it what more it needed to thrive. The garden replied that it was doing okay, but that it would be better if he spent more time enjoying it and not just looking at tasks to do. I smiled at this, because Star has often said this to me: "You could just come and sit in the garden—you do not always need to do a chore." For years I grinned and ignored her and went about my weeding and pruning, but around the same time as the ant revelations, I began to just be in the garden sometimes—listening to the birds, watching the cat, feeling the breeze, and appreciating the flowers.

The Abraham workshop was in early spring, but the weather had already turned warm and sunny. Our plum tree was beginning to bloom. I came home that afternoon and was greeted by a mass migration of ants from the house back into the garden at the exact moment I walked onto our porch. They were streaming in two sinuous parallel black rivers down the pavement of our long porch, out into the yard. They seemed to be ants purposefully moving in formation, like a marching band. I stopped and watched them, exhilarated. I called Star over to see it. Five minutes after we came home this was all done. The ants and the universe had perfectly orchestrated this loving farewell for the season. I felt honored. I felt awe. It was another lesson from the ants.

The next day was another Abraham workshop. Many participants were taking both seminars, and dozens came up to me the next day, appreciating my tale and expressing gratitude for the question. I began to get an even greater understanding of why I had been inspired to ask this question. Here was more of the process of allowing, and allowing well-being for these little ones.

A woman came up to me and related another slug story. It seems she had felt beleaguered by slugs in her San Francisco garden. She was already not a slug killer but did not know how to respond to their love of her tender vegetables. Thinking about this, she noticed an untended plot just a few doors away, with lots of healthy vegetation. She explained her concerns to the slugs and asked them if they would be willing to move down the street, to the other plot. Then she went out to do some errands. When she returned a couple of hours later, she saw a trail of slugs heading down the sidewalk from her place to the other lot. Since then, only a very few slugs have remained in her garden, and she feels friendship and kinship with these cooperative few.

A third-grade teacher approached me and said how much she had loved the story. Her classroom was full of ants, and they were constantly in and on the students' desks. Spraying pesticides had not discouraged them at all, and the teacher herself had never felt comfortable with the model of killing ants or spraying toxic chemicals around children. So they too had taken to squashing ants, which obviously didn't feel great as a teaching experience, either. She loved my experience and was eager to share what she hopes will be a lesson in interspecies cooperation with her young pupils. I asked her where would be a safe and unobtrusive location for the ants. She thought the baseboards and sidewalls of the room would be perfect. I imagine I might hear from her in the future. I hope the children come to love the ants as I do.

At lunch I sat with a number of people and again my story was discussed, together with how excited this made people feel about the possibilities. More stories of communication were shared. I talked about normal flora, and how, as I discuss in more detail later, there are more bacterial cells in and on our bodies than there are cells of what we consider to be "our body." An orchid grower sat down and we spoke about ants as well as orchids. He confirmed to me, as I had begun to suspect, that ants would take up residence in the least healthy plants. Ants are farmers, he explained, and will encourage the growth of parasitic scale. Scale now seems fine to me too, everything in its place and time. The scale further weakens the plant, which will eventually die as all things do in time, and this unwinding nourishes the life of others, as dying always fosters new growth in the eternal cycle of death and new life.

As I wrote this, a Canadian goose flew overhead, honking its approval. Canadian geese are often a personal reminder for me of synchronicity, of connectedness. Their sweeping seasonal migrations never fail to represent for me the eternal returning and renewal that is the basis of all life.

A final note to this ant story occurred throughout the next winter. It was an extended rainy season, and I kept thinking that ants would arrive en masse. I truly felt fine about their impending arrival. Eventually, a few did come but many fewer than in previous years, and they went directly to the compost bucket. The ants ventured into the trash can only a handful of times when we had put some unusually stinky stuff in there. Who could blame them? Naturally they could not resist what to them were perhaps delectable morsels. Our relationship has taken another turn. I feel genuine friendship and kinship with the ants, and feel loved and respected by them in return.

So what I learned from ants is this: Respect for all creation is a basic tenet of the language of love. It says, "I honor you, esteem you, and value your contribution to the whole. I know and appreciate your intrinsic worth." Respect implies that one will regard another with consideration for that one's autonomy. When we respect, we understand that "to everything there is a season, and a time for every purpose under heaven." There is no thing in the natural world that is inappropriate in and of itself. When we find something disagreeable, often it is our understanding that needs to be expanded, and not an external condition that needs to be changed. We cannot receive respect without offering it. Respect, like real love, is mutual.

Tools for Transformation

1. How much do you believe we can affect our experience? Is that an assumption? Have you actually tried anything else? My patients are often amazed at how easy it is to change their experience when they change the premises. They have observed

changes involving all areas of life: health, finances, job, relationships, and any life situation.

To change the premises, or your attitude, you do not need to change what is happening. In fact, you cannot change what is happening by focusing upon it. You merely need to change your thoughts about it, since thoughts lead to beliefs, beliefs form expectations, and expectations create life experience.

2. Start with something small, rather than tackling your physical health if your health is challenging for you. Instead of thinking, "I hate that there's always bad traffic on my morning commute," you could think about it a different way. You could appreciate the time it gives you to think, or find beauty in the slice of life you get to see on your route, seeing anew the clouds and trees and natural features that appear on your horizon as you travel. From this change of thoughts you might be inspired to make an audio recording of some of your favorite songs or chants and sing along, or listen to your iPod, or get books on tape/CD instead of worrying along with the news. You could get a digital voice recorder and jot down mental musings as you navigate the flow of traffic. You could make your morning commute, even if prolonged, into one of the highlights of your day.

3. If you have a health matter you are focusing upon, how are you thinking about it? Are you struggling with diabetes, fighting AIDS, combating heart disease, battling cancer? Do you see things as externally or internally generated? Do you feel invaded? If you find yourself in a struggle, which many of us do, how can you feel better right now, even before the external circumstances change at all?

4. Could you be in dialogue with the illness, on a journey with it toward finding balance? Is it possible for you to appreciate the growth that this messenger has to offer?

Not too long ago I was exploring these questions in regard to a fungus, which took up residence on my feet. By the Western model, I likely "contracted this pathogen" at a nail salon near my home. But why did this happen? While I like lovely feet, I have had questions about the sanitation of such salons, including this one. I also felt uneasy about the solvents and chemicals used for cleaning to make the place "sanitary." I have larger questions about the pedicure chemicals and the lacquers and their impact on my health and the health of other consumers and especially the health of the young, usually Asian immigrant women who work in these spas and are exposed to the fumes day after day. I had misgivings about cosmetic manufacturing and "beauty" products such as nail polishes that create a lot of ugliness in their manufacture. I have wondered about my buying in to the notion of polished nails as attractive nails, and wondered if this will eventually go the way of teeth blackening, which was cosmetically popular in upper-class society in Medieval Japan and Renaissance Europe and practiced until recently in parts of Vietnam.

I vibrationally brought all of these misgivings and contradictions to my pedicure appointments. In some ways, I am surprised I did not "contract" a fungus sooner. So now, it has been almost three years of dialogue with the fungus. It is a rich and rewarding experience, where I learn to replace small fears with love.

For two years I stopped getting pedicures but continued to care for my feet and toes. I spent a lot of time thinking about fungus as a manifestation of divinity (I am funny like that). A lot of fertile material came from that, some of which I share later in this book. I looked at pedicures playfully and found some nail products that are environmentally benign. I found a new shop for pedicures that uses environmentally friendly products and that is impeccably clean. I employed some natural and pharmaceutical products as tools while I pursued my inner explorations. I used the whole experience as an opportunity to feel better about myself, my life, fungi, and the world. I grew more relaxed, so I also stopped the worried "picking" at my cuticles that was part of the draw to pedicures in the first place. At this point, my feet look and feel fine. There is no evidence of overgrowth of fungus, and I bless the experience and the fungus for what it has taught me about interaction.

—CHAPTER FIVE—

Interrelationship: Bacteria

HEALING OCCURS IN INTERACTION BECAUSE all of physical life is lived in relationship. This is underscored from the moment of our conception. We are born as unique individuals because of a union of two individuals. We are nourished in the womb of a mother until we are ready to emerge into the world. Even after birth, we are utterly dependent upon others and will remain so throughout our lives. Human life intrinsically encompasses collaborations with other humans, physical objects, plants, animals, insects, and microbes. Relationship with thousands of elements of the natural world is required for meeting even our most basic needs for food, shelter, and warmth.

Even a hermit in a cave interacts at all moments of his physical existence: with the microflora in his body, the animals and plants that provide him nourishment, and the soil that nourishes them. He interfaces with the elements of the planet and the ecosystem that surrounds his cave; he breathes air, sits upon earth, is protected from the wind and storms by the sheltering walls of his cave. Alan Watts observed: "I'll tell you what hermits realize. If you go off into a far, far forest and get very quiet, you'll come to understand that you're connected with everything."[1]

Obviously most of us are not hermits in caves. We interact with everything our hermit does, and more. We are formed in a crucible of interrelationship, spending our lives as a part of interwoven communities. Everything we do changes us. Everything we live becomes a part of us. We are transformed at every moment, by each interaction, thought, and intention. Even the simple act of eating is an alchemical act of transformation. All foods were once tissues of other living beings. As we eat, they become us for a time, metamorphosing into blood, bone, and organs as well as emotions, concepts, and intuition.

Our lives are defined by relationships. The nature of these relationships—positive, neutral, negative—is largely up to us. As we have seen in earlier chapters, today many relationship models are available to us. The current paradigm of enmity with and dominance of the natural world is not particularly enjoyable or viable over the long term. The future pattern if we are to survive is respect, cooperation, and harmony.

We know it is possible to coexist peacefully and cooperatively with other humans and with animals. Nature and natural history provide many examples. The domestication of plant and animal species is one type of mutually cooperative endeavor. Another is non-intervention. This simply involves paying attention in our activities to avoid disturbing others, such as observing but not touching the nests of birds and turtles. Non-intervention also might involve teaching children to gaze with enjoyment and appreciation at insects, rather than reacting with fear or loathing.

There are many other relationship styles possible in which humans discover magnificent reciprocity with other species. Jane Goodall enjoyed a playful and tender camaraderie with the gorillas she studied in their native African habitat. The gardens of Findhorn in Scotland are a well-known example of a conscious collaboration between people and plants. At Findhorn, nature spirits, or devas, are partners in the creation of serene, magical gardens. In *Of Water and the Spirit*, Malidoma Somé writes of ceremonies of his people, the Dagara (in Africa), that instruct initiates in bridging worlds and co-creation with nature spirits for mutual betterment.

As the shifts in consciousness of the twenty-first century continue to unfold, we see increasing numbers of people communicating with more and more aspects of the natural world—plant, animal, and mineral. Such interactions are becoming commonplace. *The Dog Whisperer*, for example, is an incredibly popular National Geographic Channel series about Cesar Millan, a man who can communicate beautifully with dogs in their own non-verbal language. With his skills as a human-dog interpreter, Millan seems to miraculously transform vicious or maladjusted animals into friendly, happy, tractable pets.

Scientific studies have shown that talking lovingly to houseplants or playing soothing music for them promotes their growth and health.[2] The power of prayer has been examined and found to be beneficial for both the recipient and the offerer.[3] In *The Hidden Messages in Water,* Masaru Emoto details the remarkable changes in crystallized water in response to either loving or discordant thoughts and words.[4] And anyone who has ever had a "knack" for working with some other thing—whether it is a living being like a horse or a rosebush, or a physical object like a musical instrument or an automobile engine—is working in cooperative relationship.

There is nothing inherently different about our potential for interaction and benevolent relationship with microorganisms, except that they are invisible to the naked eye. The vast majority of our communication with nature is non-verbal. The first step toward any friendship is the understanding that one is possible. We are aware that humans are inextricably bonded with plants and animals. Similarly, we cannot live a day upon this planet without the cooperation of microbes. So we might want to consider liking each other and learning how collaboration feels.

Human bodies are similar to other ecosystems. Each of us is a web of interrelationships. Each individual is like a separate planet, inhabited by a myriad of species. The numbers are immense. For example, there are thousands of times more microbes in one human intestinal tract than there are galaxies in the known universe (estimated to number between two hundred billion and five hundred billion!). Right now, there are probably a thousand trillion microbes in your gut, and these contain a hundred times as many genes as the cells of your body contain.[5]

When we enjoy optimal health we are home to a myriad of other organisms: viruses, fungi, and commensal parasites. Without the supportive efforts of these busy microbes, humans could not thrive or survive. In turn, we are their universes. It is in the self-interest of all these microorganisms to nourish and support us, just as we support our health when we nurture them. The vigor and adaptability of all of us are intertwined.

There are many varieties of microorganisms on "planet person," each of which flourishes in suitable regions. This mirrors the life of various species on Earth. On the surface of the Earth, individual species require distinctive environments. Whales thrive in oceans, fungi enliven the soil, cacti flourish in the desert, and pine trees burgeon in coniferous forests. Just like on the planet's exterior, the different species of our bodies succeed in appropriate regions. Many environments found in the external world are reflected in our physical bodies.

Ocean and marsh environments teem with life. In continuous cycles, bacteria and fungi decompose organic matter into nutrients that nourish mosses, algae, and other more complex plants. These in turn feed insects and animals, that in turn feed even larger animals in a chain of interrelationship. Little fish are food for big fish. When any die, bacteria and fungi take over and the circle endlessly renews.

Terrestrial life originated in the seas and remains bound to it. Our health and vital force depend upon our internal "sea." Moisture-loving anaerobes flourish in both the marshes of our planet and the ocean of our body's intestines. The colon plays host to a mix of moisture-loving anaerobic and aerobic bacteria such as *E. coli*, bifidobacteria, and bacteroides.

Dry environments such as deserts also host a great variety of life, but life here is the sort that is best adapted to a more extreme climate. On the human body, the dry and arid regions are exterior skin surfaces. Just like in other deserts, relatively few species are found on the surface. A dry area of skin will have between one hundred and a few thousand organisms in one square centimeter (less than half an inch). This sounds like a lot, but in contrast, a square centimeter of small intestine membrane might host a billion organisms.

In the desert-like regions of our skin, most of the healthy skin bacteria are concentrated in and around sweat glands, hair follicles, and pores. Terrestrial desert dwellers congregate in cool shaded burrows just below the surface of the earth, or cluster under the shade of a mesquite bush. Hair follicles and hair itself are the "trees" of the desert regions of our skin.

The flora of the digestive tract and skin of humans and animals has been studied extensively. Nonetheless, we are only beginning to understand this complex environment. A comparison of the roles of bacteria in the marshy environment of the intestinal tract and the desert region of our skin supports understanding of ourselves as a collection of ecosystems and illustrates the level of our interdependence with microorganisms.

In a healthy intestinal tract, bacteria are plentiful. There are more bacteria in our intestinal tract than there are cells of "our" entire body. In fact, there are about ten times more of "them" than there are cells we consider to be "us." We normally harbor about four hundred types of organisms in our intestines. Some are oxygen-loving, but most are anaerobic, meaning they thrive only when oxygen is not present. This has made them challenging to study, since they die when we expose them to air. Still, they are among the most essential and prevalent of our gastrointestinal flora friends. From a human perspective, there are lots of beneficial roles for these industrious bacteria. Some of them include:

Immune support: About seventy percent of our immune system is located in the digestive tract. "Probiotic" bacteria enhance many of the functions of the immune system, acting independently as an adjunct to our cells' immune system.

Digestion and absorption of foods: The digestion of certain foods, especially carbohydrates, is facilitated by the friendly organisms of the small intestine. The foods we eat nourish their colonies. All we take in, whether food or thought, is important for determining the health of internal bacterial colonies. Each type of bacteria has its favorite diet. The kinds of bacteria most associated with vibrant health thrive upon naturally fermented foods like sauerkraut, miso, yogurt, and kefir, as well as certain fats and animal foods including saturated fats. They also require some types of fiber found in vegetables, fruits, and whole grains. They do best when we are calm, happy, and relaxed.

Barrier to pathogenic bacteria: Healthy bacteria crowd out the unwelcome visitors. When beneficial microbes that evolved along with our GI tracts colonize this region, there is not much space available for imbalanced flora to take hold. Bacteria also secrete chemical mediators that support their own species and others with whom they are harmonious. These same chemical mediators suppress bacteria that are incompatible.

Prevention of allergies: Beneficial bacteria teach the immune system to distinguish between the antigens of harmless and helpful flora and foods, and potentially dangerous ones. Allergies are a type of oversensitivity. During an allergy, the body overreacts, sensing harm in things that are not innately harmful. The presence of flourishing colonies of beneficial bacteria decreases the incidence of allergies.

Manufacture of vitamins: There is evidence that healthy forms of *E. coli* manufacture vitamin K in the human intestinal tract. In some animals, vitamin B12 is manufactured by intestinal flora. Humans, however, must consume this vitamin from animal food sources.

Elimination of toxins: Probiotic bacteria eat many of our waste products, breaking them down to component nutrients. These are recycled. What is not used is eliminated within the feces.

Stimulation of tissues: Probiotic bacteria are essential for normal development of the intestinal tract. Certain tissues like the lymphoid Peyer's patches of the intestinal tract, and the entire large intestine, require the presence of healthy bacteria for growth and maturation.

Prevention of disease: Imbalanced and reduced numbers of healthy flora are found in people with inflammatory bowel diseases like Crohn's disease and ulcerative colitis. There are also imbalances observed in most people with irritable bowel syndrome, asthma, eczema, and autoimmune illnesses.[6]

Two thousand years ago Hippocrates observed that the health of the entire body begins in the gut. Today we understand that our health is intertwined with that of the intestinal microbes. The extent to which healthy bacteria sustain our gastrointestinal health can be dramatized by just one example. It actually takes ingestion of more than ten million salmonella bacteria to sicken a healthy person or animal with good levels of supportive intestinal bacteria. But if one were artificially raised in a sterile environment, without any gastrointestinal flora, a mere **ten** bacteria would be sufficient to cause disease.[7] As our own bacteria care for us, they are providing a good home, in us, for their offspring. Our thriving means that they are fruitful and multiply.

Skin is our largest organ and the only part of the body that is fully exposed to the outside world. On our skin, different healthy bacteria such as *Staphylococcus epidermidus* and propionobacterium have a typical mutually beneficial relationship with us. From a human perspective, skin-dwelling bacteria perform many vital functions. They eat our dead skin cells and secrete a protective barrier, the acid mantle, a thin film that prevents our skin from being colonized by bacteria and fungi associated with disease. Cooperatively, the acid mantle also promotes the healthy bacteria's survival and reproduction while maintaining an ideal terrain for their offspring.

What happens when this acid mantle is disrupted? For the bacteria, it is devastating. Other organisms, including opportunistic bacteria and fungi, crowd them out, setting up conditions favorable to themselves on our skin. To us, this means skin dryness or excessive dampness, inflammation, irritation, signs of infection, pimples, broken skin, itching, flaking, and peeling. With proliferation of antibacterial soaps and cleansers, there has been a rise in serious skin infections.

These cleansers not only kill imbalanced and disease-causing flora, they destroy the wholesome and industrious healthy bacteria. Without them, we have no acid mantle and are much more vulnerable to skin infection and inflammation.

This brief examination indicates one way that we are utterly dependent upon microscopic life for our very existence. But most scientific studies of microbes are directed at understanding what will kill them. Even looking at normal flora, many studies warily consider under what conditions these benefactors will become destructive. Wanting to destroy something does not lead to a spirit of cooperation, harmony, or understanding. We need much more comprehension of how the lives of microbes interact mutually with the lives of people and animals. It may be hubris to believe we can proclaim some microbes beneficial and others hazardous. We "wipe out" one microbe, like smallpox, and hundreds of other, more "virulent" organisms come rushing in to fill the gap. Nature fills a vacuum. Destruction of living organisms, and even microorganisms, by poisoning, burning, starving, or attacking in the name of "science" is not born of a science rooted in positive relationship. It is not the science of love. It is a disconnected science. Cooperative relationship is not achieved through hate. Living beings including humans, ants, and microbes will share their secrets with those they love and have come to trust.

It is not too late to change the path we are on. Instead of exploitation, there can and must be a relationship of mutual caring and respect, underscored by a knowledge of mutual interdependence, for all parties to flourish. I encourage the medical and scientific world to consider these concepts as we formulate more science born of a framework of relationship. The reference compounds of all life on this planet are DNA and RNA. We share these compounds with every known living thing—streptococci and walnuts, paramecia and sunflowers, mice and chimpanzees. At a more basic cosmological level, all matter is made of the same atoms and subatomic particles. While each being is unique, we are all interrelated at the most minute molecular and atomic level.

We need to understand the web of life woven around us. We need ways to study life while honoring life. If we assume a position of trust and benevolence, then we might consider that an overgrowth or imbalance of any species in our personal ecosystem may have information for us about the balance in our life. We can form a relationship with any and all beings. It is in our relationships that we will be transformed.

One of my favorite discoveries in researching this chapter was finding a website detailing a body of artwork called "The Normal Flora Project." This is an ongoing area of exploration for artist Anna Dumitriu, whose undertaking has had many manifestations. She has worked with culturing normal flora of various environments and then photographing them, and creating sculptures from her images. Her oeuvre includes communicating with bacteria in their own language of biochemistry, and a project linking bacteria with cutting-edge digital technology. Dumitriu is fascinated by the vast interconnectivity of microbial life of the globe. She points out that most bacteria are neither "friendly" nor "evil," as they are portrayed in the media. "Bacteria," she says, "are mostly just there." She also writes, "There are more bacteria living on the end of your finger than there are people in the world." Dumitriu combines a childlike curiosity with a mystic's sensitivity and an artist's finesse. Her works are exhibited widely, and she has collaborated extensively with medical students, scientists, and other artists. She has developed playful and loving tools to visualize, appreciate, and enjoy the usually unseen realms of microbial life.[8]

Tools for Transformation

1. Try interacting with bacteria, maybe those that are in your body right now. Talk to them with respect, explain your current situation, and tell them what you need. Express your

desire for cooperation, and your willingness to acknowledge their divinity. Microbes were here long before people and have ancient wisdom. This conversation can all be in your imagination, as, of course, the real communication is non-verbal. Be attentive and yet easy about it.

Try the interaction after meditation or an activity that helps you to feel centered and aligned. You are unlikely to get good information or a sense of communication when you are angry, tired, or frustrated. Choose a time when you are refreshed and relaxed and have time to play with the exercise.

A sample interaction with a bacteria such as Lyme *(Borrelia burgdorferi)* might go like this:

You: Hi, Lyme spirochetes. I've never talked with microbes before, but since you decided to live here in my body for a while, I thought it was a good time to start.

(Feel/listen for greeting from them; this may be a feeling or a sensation.)

You: I notice from my collection of symptoms and some medical tests that you have taken up residence in my body. I am wondering, "Why me? What do you like about my body?" (Ask if you are interested in knowing this or believe it is relevant, otherwise just move on to the next question.)

(Listen internally for response.)

You: I recently began wondering about our relationship. I know we got off to a bad start with me taking drugs to kill you and me believing that you were making me feel sick. Now I'd like to change that. I took that action because I was afraid, but I now have a glimmer of a different understanding. Recently, I've begun to see there is something futile in this. Also I've noticed that your kind live in lots of people and animals, and many of those people feel well even though your kind live in them. The reason I was trying to kill you is just because I felt sick and wanted to be well. I have lately been thinking that perhaps you are not my enemy. I am now realizing that I have no need to hate or fear you. I just want to feel well, healthy, and strong.

(Feel/listen for response.)

There is plenty of room for all of us to live and thrive. Do you think we can come up with a new relationship that we can agree upon?

(Feel/listen for response.)

Right now I'm feeling foggy-headed, tired, and my joints hurt almost all the time. Can you help me feel better with that?

(Feel/listen.)

I think that as I feel better and happier in my body, my body will feel better to you too. I believe we can find a nice balance, along with the rest of my bacteria friends. There is room enough for everyone to feel good. Do you agree? Feel free to talk to me about anything!

(Feel/listen.)

I've enjoyed this interaction immensely. I plan to continue to work at hearing and understanding you, and I hope this is the beginning of a beautiful co-creative friendship. Thanks!

Periodically pause to listen for response. Write down any impressions that may come to you from this dialogue, even if you think you are making it up.

2. Eventually try to write your own dialogue and questions based upon what you want to know. This is a process of developing relationship, not a one-time deal. Make agreements with the microbes that are comfortable to you and then keep your word. Don't pretend to be friendly—admit any fears and concerns you might have. The natural world responds to your vibration, your energetic output, not your words. Words are a

way for *you* to focus attention. The natural world understands vibration, intention, and thought forms. You may sense actual words as a response, which is great, but it is good to understand that words are an interpretation of the communication.

Microbes may ask you for things—dietary changes, more rest, more fun, less worry, greater self-esteem, more stretching or exercise, and more contact with nature. Play with this. This is a simple yet revolutionary approach that can lead to experiencing a new kind of health and an inner transformation.

—CHAPTER SIX—

On Conscious Co-Creation

THE GOLDEN RULE STATES, "Do unto others as you would have others do unto you." Consider instead that a more accurate statement of the Golden Rule is "What we do to others, we do to ourselves." There is a relationship between our thoughts, intentions, and actions and the outcomes we achieve. What we focus upon we attract to ourselves.

For the last two thousand years, most of us have thought of human "others" when considering the Golden Rule. But the universe does not distinguish among types of others. The emotion of hatred is always detrimental to us, whether it is directed at "terrorists," our neighbor whose new house addition is blocking our view, the swarm of flies buzzing around our head, or Lyme spirochetes in our bloodstream. We are never enriched by hatred and fear. They diminish us because they magnify our illusion of separation.

Love, on the other hand, amplifies the best in us. It makes us whole. Love for our pets, a lavish spring garden, a butterfly alighting on a blossom, or a star-filled sky is not different from love for our fiancé, our child, or ourselves. Love is always life-affirming and deeply sustaining.

Our emotions affect us and not others—whether we are feeling love or fear. Love is deeply nourishing. Like oxygen, it is essential for life. The emotions of hatred and fear are poisons that literally stop us in our tracks. They paralyze us, physically halting energy production at a cellular level. We are not meant to hate.

What we feel shapes us emotionally and becomes interwoven and stored in our physical body. The sum of how we feel, act, and react through the stream of moments is our creation of life. It is the painting that we paint, the book that we write. Each chapter, each word, is written in present time. As we create our life we create our physical and emotional health, or lack thereof. It is the soul, the inner being, that forms the body as life is lived.

At the height of the Cold War, it was fashionable and encouraged to fear and hate Communists. Contemporary propaganda today encourages Americans to fear and hate "Muslim extremists." The arguments are mind-numbingly similar: "They are out to destroy our way of life, they are sneaky, we can't trust them." Us/them, us/them, us/them.

Even those who may not consider themselves prejudiced believe it is acceptable to fear and hate snakes, spiders, rats, and cockroaches as well as viruses, bacteria, and cancers. People fear and hate their own fat. But fear and hate are mentally and emotionally toxic. Us/them exists only in our minds. Our dichotomizations damage only ourselves.

Grace can be described as a direct communication heard, received, and incorporated. It fundamentally alters our perception as well as the course of our life. Grace is an experience of knowing. It may feel like it comes from outside ourselves, and many religions seemingly teach that premise. But grace can be cultivated. Grace thrives in fertile and tended soil. Grace arrives when receptivity is there, when desire, openness, or faith is strong. Grace comes when we plant ourselves firmly in our heart and dedicate ourselves to hearing and responding to its truth.

The radio show *This American Life* broadcast a presentation of a true story entitled "Heretics," which first aired on December 7, 2008. This story is relevant to our current discussion of dichotomization and co-creation, and is available as a podcast on the Chicago Public Radio/*This American Life* website.[1] It tells the story of a popular evangelical minister, the Reverend Carlton Pearson. Here's my synopsis of this inspiring biographical program:

Reverend Pearson is a prominent evangelical Christian minister. A powerful and charismatic speaker, he was, for many years, the protégé of Oral Roberts, who considered him his "African-American son." Reverend Pearson's reputation and fiery style helped him build a huge congregation in Tulsa, Oklahoma. Pearson was always a deep thinker. He believed he received an epiphany from God after seeing a televised program about suffering people in Rwanda, who his church taught were going to hell because they were not already Christians. This moment of grace led Reverend Pearson to the inescapable conclusion that he did not believe in hell. He could only see the logic in a God of love. After this revelation he no longer believed that God despised non-Christians or homosexuals, because God does not despise. God loves. God is not to be feared and God does not punish. Instead he came to believe that we punish ourselves when we remove ourselves from the love that is God.

Reverent Pearson changed his message, based upon this revelation, and in the process lost ninety-five percent of his congregation, who were not ready for the message of the love of God. This brings to mind the adage that "the only thing more surprising than a non-Christian is a true Christian." Those who remained in his congregation saw a transformation. Pearson now preaches of the love of God. Today, all are welcome under his broad and loving umbrella.

A Course in Miracles teaches something similar. We create hell for ourselves, here on Earth, when we voluntarily, and perhaps unknowingly, separate ourselves from God's love. Fear holds us apart from the true love that is God. Our experience of heaven or hell in life is dependent upon our perspective. We are all children of God, exactly as we are. We are reflections of God's great love. We are God-essence. It is our illusion of separation that creates pain. Pain is not reality. Separating ourselves from our divine essence is the cause of pain.

As divine beings, part of a universal oneness and eager participants in a human life stream, we co-create with others. Others with whom we interact are fundamentally interrelated with us. Co-creation, like relationship, is inevitable as we move through life experience. Conscious co-creation is a choice. We interact and co-create in every moment of our existence. But it is entirely up to each of us whether co-creation is done with awareness and intent, or whether we just drift through our lives reacting to whatever is in front of us.

"The Law of Attraction" is one premise that explains the concept of conscious co-creation. Throughout the ages and continuing today, many teachers offer variations on this theme, some couched in mysticism, others quite blatantly and openly.

Two concepts related to the Law of Attraction are "Our thoughts create reality" and "We create our own personal reality through our thoughts." Our focus, beliefs, and intentions are the engine that drives us toward what we attract. As individuals, our perceptions and beliefs form the fabric of our experiences. As groups, society, and mass consciousness, our collective beliefs gather momentum driving toward experience in civilizations.

While the concepts of the Law of Attraction and creating one's own reality are much bandied about, they can be difficult at first to wrap one's mind around. Clearly most people do not seem to be creating the experience they desire. Often, quite the opposite is true. Wars, illnesses, and suffering are all present in the world, and few if any actually desire these. If we in fact create our own reality with our thoughts, why is there so much suffering in the world? In addition, many people have believed in things that were later proved to be incorrect.

Creating our reality is usually not done consciously, though it can be a conscious process. Instead, most people have been trained by culture to focus willy-nilly upon whatever is in front of them, desired or undesired. So, in effect, they create more of the same. Our power of focus is what determines our power of creation. If we focus on what worries us, what we believe is wrong, and what we observe in our immediate environment, whether or not it is remotely like anything we desire, then the world mirrors that back to us. In the Abraham-Hicks vernacular this is called "creating by default." I witness default creation constantly among my patients, friends, and family. I see the ways that I have created by default. When I think I am not good enough, I do not take attractive opportunities as they are presented to me. If I believe I am too fat, I give the cells and organs of my body a message to remain in that condition, upholding my belief. If many of our cultural cues and thoughts are fearful, we create with fear and what we experience is scary, and not what we desire. Creating from fear and hate only engenders more fear and hate. A way out of that cycle is to learn to create with love.

Beliefs relate to how life is experienced. The Law of Attraction gathers thoughts of a similar nature. If we believe the Earth is flat, we will find others who accept that as a fact. If we believe something fervently, we can find much corroborating evidence, even if that is not the way it actually is. Our belief does not make the Earth flat, but it makes it extremely unlikely that we will be the intrepid explorer who goes out and discovers something different. People who believe that God hates are easily able to find others who confirm this opinion. We find new evidence and new revelations only when we doubt prevailing beliefs and only when we are open-minded.

I have consciously worked with the Law of Attraction for many years. Once I understood clearly that we create the reality we experience via our thoughts, beliefs, and expectations, my only job was to get happy and truly expect desired outcomes. This is, of course, an evolving process. It may sound simplistic but is not. While it might seem easy to always select what is more joyous, we know that life is more complicated. Even though the goal is to feel better, it requires active attention. It also requires not digging deeper into things that feel bad, even though that may seem tempting or "true". Thoughts similar to the ones we are already thinking, whether pleasing or depressing, are easiest to find by the Law of Attraction. So in many ways it is simpler, but far less satisfying, to just stay where we already are. Yet consciously shifting thoughts and actions toward greater harmony results in tangible positive benefits. I have observed in patients, friends, and myself that as more thoughts are loving and joyous, we create a better and better life experience, improved health, and overall well-being.

Fortunately, it is pleasant to learn to create with love and joy because love is natural to us. Love is what we are born for. Look at babies and small children. They are gleeful, wanting play, physical affection, nourishment, and joy. Children inspire those feelings in others. How many times have the images of laughing babies delighted you? How often do you see new parents performing hysterical antics just to elicit a smile or chuckle from their child? Everyone around is enlivened by the interaction.

Co-creation implies consciousness. If we are co-creating with another, it would indicate to us that there is some measure of consciousness in the other. Most of us accept that many if not all animals have consciousness. Clearly we co-create with our pets. They have specific needs and desires that they express to us. There is a big difference between the way my dog Lily conveys to me that she wants a walk and how she demonstrates that she'd like some of my steak. But she, like most dogs, is a happy-go-lucky pooch and will accept a walk or tug session easily, instead of the steak.

Many animals are intelligent and self-aware. Parrots approach the intelligence and language skills of a five-year-old child. Chimpanzees and other higher primates like bonobos can learn to understand simple conversation. They even display some amount of reasoning in decision-making. Raccoons, as anyone who has dealt with them knows, are crafty, and rats will cooperate with one another to solve complex tasks like opening a trash can full of food.

But what about consciousness in bacteria, fungi, viruses, and spirochetes or in particles such as electrons, protons, neutrons, and even

tinier particles like hadrons and quarks? Could they have consciousness as well? And if so, what sort would it be? Could we interact with
it? Consciousness in inanimate matter seems the most unlikely to us,
but that is exactly what quantum physics requires. Remember that it
is the presence of an observer that determines if a photon is a wave or
a particle. Until an observer is present to observe any iota of matter,
it exists in superposition, undetermined, both a particle and a wave.
In superposition it is as if the photon is in the doorway between non-
physical and physical reality. It is not yet fully manifest as what it will
be. It is potential. The photon's state in subsequent physical reality is
determined only after an observer is present to observe it. This implies that even at the level of elementary particles, somehow the photon must have awareness that it is being observed. It must somehow
be aware of the relationship it has with the observer.

A difference is felt on the minutest level from the application of
mind. Within this universe we participate in the creative process. Material reality, while seemingly solid in appearance, is actually a vibratory dance mediated by the mind. The existence of physical matter is
determined by consciousness. We can learn to love all our creations
as we come to see they are parts of ourselves since we are the minds
that observe, think, and create.

As a health-care practitioner and healer, I find the work of helping
others to love and accept their own co-creations the most fascinating
and challenging. Healing occurs as we collect the missing, rejected,
and neglected pieces of ourselves. We learn first to accept and then to
love them. For example, a patient I'll call "Lara" consulted with me
about her arthritis, back pain, and skin problems. In the interview she
had a long list of ways she was not good enough. She summed this up
by saying that she knows she is "bad at taking care of herself." Her mea
culpa included eating an excessive amount of sweets that are "not
good for her" and "not exercising or stretching enough," even though
stretching seems to help her joints. She was ashamed that she spends

"way too much time playing video games." All through our consult, she repeatedly judged herself harshly. She felt she was "ugly" because she had gained weight and considered herself too fat. Her weight gain was affecting her marriage as, surprise, surprise, her husband was now critical of her appearance as well, and he agreed that she had poor self-control. Mostly, Lara demonstrated to me that she was judge, jury, and executioner.

Lara's husband probably had little awareness of Lara's role in their marital co-creation of his critical feelings and remarks. He undoubtedly observed her repeatedly complaining about her weight and expressing her feelings of powerlessness to change. Lara was unconsciously programming him to believe precisely what she did not want him to think, but what she herself believed.

The human brain contains many structures that facilitate the acquisition of language and the assimilation of cultural cues. These include mirror neurons, structures in the frontal lobes of the brain. These neurons respond identically when we perform an action and when we see someone else doing it. These neurons "mirror" the behaviors of others to us as if these actions were our own.[2] Many parents, for example, will feed their baby and instinctively open their own mouth as they do so, mirroring the expected action to the baby. We see and hear words and behaviors in someone else, and our brain interprets this as if we experienced it ourselves. Such structures help maintain culturally coherent associations between our external observations and what are currently socially appropriate responses and actions. So, through her words and actions, Lara was giving her husband daily cues about the culture of their home that essentially said: "Don't respect me, don't think I am attractive."

Mirror neurons also assist us with the "rehearsal effect." When we practice doing something in our mind, our physiology responds as if we were doing it actively. The more clearly we can visualize an activity, the more physically real it is to us. The muscles of a runner running a race in his mind will twitch and fire. A person recovering from a spinal cord injury plays the sequence of walking and standing many times over in her mind on the road to recovery. In using osteopathic work and Ortho-Bionomy®, I often ask a patient to imagine performing an activity. The patient's muscles engage as if he were actually doing the task. Using this tool, I can understand how the patient uses his body in movement while he is in fact lying on the table. The rehearsal effect is augmented as more of the mind is involved. Imaging something, complete with the emotions we might feel, enhances the physiologic effects and the patterning we are offering to our consciousness.

Initially Lara was not ready for the message I offered. She tried to enlist me in agreement that she was much too fat, though by most standards she's only a little chubby, perhaps twenty pounds over the book-value ideal weight. Several times during our interview she said that she couldn't be happy unless she loses weight but feels powerless to do so. So she was effectively saying that she cannot be happy. Lara was hoping I would find a medical problem, perhaps an undetected thyroid problem, that would help her change this unhappy condition. While I certainly was willing to do whatever medical work-up was appropriate, I suspected the problem was in her thoughts and not her endocrine system. Her pervasive low self-esteem and self-criticism gave her a body that reflected her dissatisfaction with herself.

What is the role of others in my, your, or Lara's co-creation of life? In some ways, others are on their own trajectories, independently experiencing their own lives in unique ways. But in relationship, others mirror and amplify us to ourselves by their presence and our interactions.

I have observed that those I admire the most are a little ahead of me, being aspects of the self I am inside. They are externalizing possibilities for me, showing me the way to be more of what I desire to be. When we admire others, we are more than halfway there.

Similarly, those that most annoy and confound us mirror ways we are still growing. They amplify parts of ourselves that we have made into the Other. They remind us of our shadows—aspects of ourselves that we reject. This is why so many spiritual teachings focus on forgiveness. We are really forgiving ourselves when we forgive others. The external world seems separate from us, but the only way we experience it is in the dark, silent recesses of our mind and in the stillness of our heart.

What we say matters to the heart of us. It matters to our emotional and physical health. Usually we do not examine our words too deeply. Cultural forces largely determine what we commonly say. Our peers, our families, what we have observed and what others have told us to believe form our expectations.

As we looked lovingly at each of her issues over subsequent visits, Lara was slowly able to understand how they came about, and to let go of self-judgments. She noticed that her arthritis flared up when she felt angry but did not express herself. When she first visited, Lara was a "nice" person and not in touch with her feelings of anger. She had many challenging experiences in her past. Her body developed a pattern that put the anger into her joints. Arthritic pain came when her emotions were congested and dammed up. During the course of our treatments, Lara began to stretch regularly and also to express feelings more honestly, both to herself and the others around her.

Lara also noticed that by believing herself to be fat and unattractive, she had neglected simple things like smiling and laughing, things that make anyone more attractive. She looked in the mirror and saw that she was beginning to get frown lines. She decided it was worthwhile to try to change her thoughts. As part of this, she realized that she is no longer a twenty-something and perhaps some curves are nice. As Lara began to see herself as sexy, not surprisingly her husband started to see her the same way. As I suspected, she did not have a thyroid problem, though she did have some mineral imbalances contributing to her skin condition. We corrected those with dietary changes and a few months of nutritional supplements.

In an ideal medical appointment, the patient—and at times, her family members—co-create health solutions with the health care professional. The patient is a whole person and is treated as such. The complex web of interactions contributing to the current situation is evaluated. All relevant aspects of the patient's physical, emotional, and spiritual state are part of the discussion. With the bigger picture in mind, a plan evolves that includes the expertise and assessment of the physician as well as the unique circumstances of each patient.

For example, in my practice I often recommend dietary changes to patients. This can be an appropriate first step for shifting, giving patients a feeling of control and an opportunity for self-care. In a few patients, though, especially those with a history of eating disorders, dietary changes can dramatically increase anxiety and stress, triggering new problems. For these patients, other changes such as breathing techniques, exercise prescription, and herbal or nutritional supplements have a larger role. Occasionally I have met patients who, although they deeply desire health, resist any programmatic change. That is okay too. The role of a holistic practitioner, as I see it, is to work with patients where they are at, empowering and soothing. One of my teachers, the distinguished Chinese medicine scholar and writer Ted Kaptchuk, OMD, said in class that the patient should begin to feel better while sitting in the office, before any needles are placed or herbal prescription filled. His words have been incorporated into every day of my life as a physician.

As I came to understand co-creation and the role thoughts play in our physical and emotional health, it was clear to me why Dr. Kaptchuk's words were so significant. How a patient feels in the office interaction sets the stage for the unfolding of healing. As a physician, if I can be optimistic about a prognosis for health and can embody that vision while interacting with my patient, then the patient is working with someone who sees and mirrors his or her health. A milieu of well-being is created. I maintain the knowledge of health's surety while the patient takes the appropriate steps to catch up to the vision.

As with a series of medical visits, reading a book is a co-creation. There is a script followed by writers and readers. Normally books are written by first setting up "the problem." Current undesirable conditions are examined in great detail, so readers can get a clear picture of every nuance the writer perceives is wrong. Theoretically, this common strategy sets the stage for an author to provide a contrasting viewpoint. The existing situation is the proverbial "straw man" to be knocked down by the superiority of the new perspective. But while some juxtaposition of the old and new can be helpful for appreciating fresh concepts, in my experience focusing extensively on problems is not empowering either to the reader or the writer. Examination of a problem is useful merely as a point of clarification. A prolonged negative discourse mires people in a state of fear about the current dire circumstances instead of anchoring them in optimism about new perspectives.

Focus on problems can prevent the "ah-ha!" moment of the solution from coming forward. One famous Einstein quote addresses this: "The problems that exist in the world today cannot be solved by the level of thinking that created them." I experience the truth of these words often, even in contemplating my writing. When I trudge and drudge, little comes. Doing so, I feel frustrated and exhausted. My best tactic is to pose a question to myself, then go off and do something else. Occasionally I do this for days until, in a moment of ease, everything clarifies and coalesces. The solution comes to me while gardening, during a hike in nature, or even awakening me in the middle of the night. I savor these moments of epiphany and over time have released the feeling of scarcity about them coming. Insights are as abundant as the ease that I allow myself. We all need harmony, rest, and peace of mind for new visions and solutions to percolate. New perceptions come over and over again from a calm center.

Nature, the universe with the divine love underlying all, is rooting for us. Even while we are writing and reading, we can imagine and dream together, beginning the process of co-creation of our splendid future anchored in knowledge of divine love. This strategy changes our momentum and direction of focus. When we focus on what we want and start envisioning it in any group, including a group of readers, we participate constructively in what has been termed "the group mind." Another term for the group mind is "the noosphere," a word coined by the twentieth-century French Jesuit mystic Pierre Teilhard de Chardin.

Demonstrations of the effects of a group mind have been explored scientifically. Experiments indicate that groups of people focusing together change consciousness. There are approximately seventy-five universities and labs worldwide participating in a long-term study of the effects of mass focus upon random number generators, computer applications that randomly select and display numbers every few moments. It is fascinating to note that the random number selections repeatedly become non-random and exhibit coherence when enough people in proximity to a number generator focus together upon the same thing.[3] This can be a news event like the OJ Simpson trial, or the tragic events of the Indonesian or Japanese tsunamis, or even your local team winning the Super Bowl.

Our visions and common focus together can manifest a better future. They help us perceive the current situation in the best possible light. When we see the cup half full, we are empowered to explore better scenarios. The silver lining in that which is less desirable is the inspiration for creation of something new and wonderful.

This book is an exercise in demonstrating the power and fun of working consciously with the Law of Attraction to deliberately create a desired shared reality. I envision what feels delicious and beautiful to me, and I invite readers to do the same. We can weave the unique contributions of each of our dreams into the mix. I encourage readers to co-create a new viewpoint and to coin new loving words and send them forth into the world. Although each of us has a unique viewpoint, we agree on many things when we proceed from a heart-centered perspective. We all want well-being, joy, beauty, health, satisfaction, material comfort, and pleasure for ourselves and for others. We can dream a dream of our world together and make it so.

There are no enemies because, in the words of Walt Kelly's comic strip character Pogo: "We have met the enemy and he is us." If an enemy shows up on our doorstep, we have invited him there to play the role of the enemy. We have long lived with an ideology that sets up the "Other" as one to be feared, mistrusted, conquered, hated, and destroyed. The Other may be our neighbor, or bacteria, or terrorists, or another nation, or "bad" extraterrestrials (aliens), or "the devil," or our parents, or drugs, or even our own frailties. It may be a generic "evil" or "pestilence." The net result of all this fear and hatred is more fear and hatred. We see environmental destruction, wars, cruelty to animals, prejudice, and intolerance promoted in an ongoing Orwellian drama.

Frankly, I am bored with the repetitive war, the ongoing cycle of hate and fear promoted by the current cultural model. You probably are too, since you are reading this book. People are beginning to notice that the same actions yield the same results. We are growing up and waking up, recognizing that we have been exploring a bad dream of our own design, like repeatedly choosing to go to scary movies and be terrified over and over again. We have allowed ourselves to forget that we are in a scary movie, and we began to confuse it with our external "reality," doubting whether there is anything beyond this tired melodrama.

The greater part of us—our soul, higher self, or inner being (take your pick on terminology)—knows and has always known that this illusion is our own creation. We can regard our current situation as a complex puzzle, a cosmic Rubik's cube that we invented and tasked ourselves with solving. As a human race, we are closing in on the solution. If you have ever watched *Star Trek*, it is as if we have just begun to recognize that we are living in a limited holodeck program and getting bored with the belief systems that perpetuate this particular illusion.

In my late teens I encountered the works of Jane Roberts and Seth. The simple phrase "you create your own reality" was a lightning bolt for me, illuminating a pivotal understanding that rang so true in my heart that I built much of my subsequent life upon it. Gradually, I no longer believed in random events outside my control. Even if I could not immediately see how I, via thoughts and beliefs, had generated an encounter, I understood that it was mine and began to take credit for it, and to enjoy the resulting empowerment.

As we awaken to our greater consciousness, we come to a deeper understanding that love is the fabric underlying all existence. Love calls this universe into being, weaving the threads of physical reality into the astounding tapestry of life. There is no part, immense or tiny, that is excluded from love. The universe presents itself to us in a hall of mirrors. We co-create with others in a dance orchestrated by our souls. We are waking to our wonders, and a collective conscious awareness is stirring.

TOOLS FOR TRANSFORMATION

1. *Observing your heart*

   I have spent a lot of time examining my heart. This is an ongoing process that involves perceiving the physical structure (the beating heart) as well as the emotional/spiritual organ. I have noticed that every emotion I feel resonates in my heart. I have painstakingly tracked my emotions: the ones that feel good such as love, fulfillment, and wonder, and those that feel not so good such as anger, fear, and worry. Each of them resonates physically in my heart.

There is much to be gained by such examination. It can become a great habit. I perceive that for me, upsetting emotions, particularly fear, have spiny and pointy shapes. Recurrent fears feel like huge spikes. The energy released as these are dissolved is enormous. I once painted the energy pattern I saw as an old "issue" became comet-like in its positive power of transformation.

I have found that stock phrases such as "from the bottom of my heart" have actual meaning. The bottom of my heart is the seat of my deepest and longest-held feelings. My heart is only ever "full" from a deep sense of well-being, appreciation, or gladness. My heart feels empty or depleted when I feel isolated, lonely, or despairing. Anger "stabs me in the heart." Agitation feels like incoherence throughout my heart. My heart "overflows" when I feel my connection to the divine within me; and as I strengthen and breathe, filling myself with the strength of that connection, I can radiate that feeling to others.

When I am at a loss as to what more to do for a patient, I simply listen without judgment and silently offer my heartfelt connection to peace. From that space, often, the perfect words or question will come to me to coax the individual toward wellness. Sometimes they just feel a sense that a lifeline of quiet comfort is available to them. Often patients tell me that something I said to them years ago was a profound turning point in their lives. I feel truly blessed to participate co-creatively in this manner.

2. To begin watching your heart, gently settle into your breathing. Let go of thoughts; allow them to drift away like wispy clouds. Breathe into your heart and out, as in prior tools. When you are calm, it is time to deliberately introduce thoughts and emotions to see where they go in your heart and your body.

First, notice if your words and thoughts "strike" you. Does that have a sensation? Do different thoughts impact you differently? When you observe or consider something pleasing, find it in your heart. Do the same for experiences that are upsetting. Notice what shape, texture, and size your thoughts and experiences have as they come into the heart field. Do they have colors? Does anything happen with your heart rate or your comfort level when you track various thoughts and experiences to your heart? Notice if thoughts and experiences track to other areas of your body. Find the connection between those areas and your heart.

Make notes, record sounds, or draw pictures of what comes to you.

When you are done, return to your peaceful, centered breathing. Let your heart know that you are interested in clearer, gentler, and subtler modes of communication.

—CHAPTER SEVEN—
Maps of the Worlds

I MAGINE THAT THE NATURAL WORLD is always communicating with us, whether or not we consciously understand the messages. Like the Inuit who have so many words to perceive and describe snow, there are many ways for each of us to process information from both our inner and outer worlds. In contemporary society, we do not have commonly used language to describe huge parts of the informational exchange that is constantly occurring. Instead we have been culturally programmed to ignore the communications of the natural world, since no words in common parlance are available to mediate the interaction. The very existence of these modes of communication has been largely forgotten in "modern" Western civilization.

In the scientific community, people who speak of the immanence of nature, or of any aspect of the natural world communicating directly with them or others, are generally belittled, ridiculed, or ignored. These tactics, typical of bullying, are all parts of the spectrum of a war mentality. The more oppressive the regime, the less tolerant it is of nonconformity. In our culture, a sense of the presence of nature is "allowed" in the arts and literature, but it is usually rejected in "science." The arts are a mode of self-expression, while science is supposedly "objective."

Claims of objectivity functionally squelch freedom of expression and exploration of subjective experience. Even well-done scientific studies that look at the inter-communication of individuals and aspects of the natural world, or telepathic connections between humans, are summarily dismissed by the reigning hierarchy or labeled as "soft science." In science today we find a situation of smug stagnation, similar to that of the Middle Ages in Europe, wherein only certain condoned ways of viewing reality are accepted. The unfortunate consequence of this limited worldview has been a dearth of technologies that are in harmony with nature. Since scientists believe it is not possible to hear or interact with the voice of nature, they ignore and deny that there is anything to listen to.

Science did not evolve this way accidentally. There was, in fact, a deliberate exclusion of any matters divine or spiritual in the development of contemporary science. This was not in order to be more "objective." There was a more interesting and calculated reason that the conjoined twins of spirit and science were separated at the birth of modern science. To understand the roots of our current dilemma, and how to set sail into a more expanded realm of communication, it is helpful to examine what was going on when modern science was in its early stages. To do so requires a brief survey of some philosophical and religious concepts such as Materialism, Scientism, Dualism, and Monism, as well as a quick glance at seventeenth-century European politics.

Materialism and Scientism

Materialism, a dominant theme in contemporary civilization, is the view that physical matter is the only reality. Many well-meaning, humanitarian people believe in this viewpoint, without any knowledge of its (ironically) theological roots. According to this philosophy, all observable things and processes can be understood and explained as manifestations of existing material substance. In other words, to Materialism, everything that IS comes from things that already exist physically.

Scientism, the child of materialism, is a religious-like belief in the power of science to understand and know all things. Scientism claims that it is always possible to understand the cause of anything, purely from that which already exists physically. The religiosity comes in as people believe, in the face of contradictory evidence, that it is possible for Materialist science to understand all things without taking into account the non-physical.

Many people are not aware that Scientism and Materialism are strains of thought unique to Western philosophy. Traditional Asian thought is based in Idealism. A central tenet of Idealism is that non-physical reality is primary and that physical reality is an extension from the non-physical. This thinking is not entirely foreign to Western thought, as Plato posited the same concept more than two thousand years ago.

Materialism could be said to have two parents. One is the philosophical idea of a mind-body split promoted by seventeenth-century French philosopher René Descartes. The second parent of Materialistic science was the preface of a book, dedicated to King Charles II as representative of the Church of England, by Thomas Sprat of the Royal Society of England.

Descartes, Monism, and Dualism

Dualism is a philosophical viewpoint with important ramifications for contemporary civilization. In dualistic thinking there is always a division between two types of substances or behaviors. Juxtapositions of good and evil, sacred and profane, light and dark, subject and object are all examples of dualistic concepts. Dualism contrasts with Monism, where there is an underlying unity despite the appearance of diversity. Monistically, there is ultimately only one greater reality, the sacred or divine, and everything in material reality flows from it and always connects with it. Monism is the wellspring viewpoint of most religions, including the Western religions Judaism, Christianity, and Islam as well as major Eastern religions including Buddhism, Hinduism, and Zoroastrianism.

Whatever is at their core, however, most religions today are more dualistic in their practical applications. In day-to-day teachings, theological and doctrinaire disagreements between religious sects cloud appreciation of any underlying unity. Today, Monism's potentially practical applications are functionally obscured by idiosyncrasies of theology. People are not encouraged to think along these lines, despite the core understanding of our oneness. Monistically, for example, we would of course "love our neighbor as our self" because we would recognize that ultimately our neighbor *is* our self. In Monistic thinking, there is a single greater reality that encompasses this material reality. What we experience as physical reality, our reality of apparent phenomena, is just a subset of a greater unity.

Doctrinaire pronouncements, even of religious factions, are a form of dualism. If we are all one, all flowing from the eternal divine, then my God is not greater than your God, and my way is not better than your way, because there is not my God and your God. Monism versus dualism has a long history in Western philosophical thought, stretching back to ancient Greeks. This book is a product of a Monistic understanding.

René Descartes was a brilliant mathematician and philosopher born in 1596, a dualist best known for the statement: "I think, therefore I am." This conclusion led him to the idea of a mind-body split. Descartes believed that the mind and matter were two separate and distinct substances belonging to two distinct and virtually unconnected realms. To Descartes, mind thinks and is entirely non-physical, while matter exists entirely in physical space. In his dualistic concept, the mind and soul are non-physical and do not influence matter, since all physical objects are ruled by unchangeable principles of physics. In Descartes's cosmology, or understanding of the universe, the mind communicates with the body only at the pineal gland.

Descartes had many other notions that have long ago been disproved and rejected. For example, he believed that only humans feel pain, and advocated and performed experimentation on live animals without anesthesia. Nonetheless, his mind-body split theory has persisted in some circles until today, largely because of a theological snafu.

Ironically, materialism in science was born in a turf-dividing concession to seventeenth-century Western religious and political institutions. The seventeenth century in England was a turbulent period. Much of the fighting evolved from religious disputes. A series of civil wars extended from 1642 to 1651. One of the major precipitating factors of these wars was a growing hostility concerning disagreements about questions of theology and liturgy in the Church of England. King Charles I married a French Roman Catholic, Henrietta-Maria de Bourbon, shortly after he assumed the throne in 1625. Many Protestant English were alarmed that a Catholic prince might inherit the throne. This became a flashpoint that inflamed other political tensions of the era. Charles I was eventually executed in 1649, and his son, Charles II, though a Protestant, was sent into exile. Oliver Cromwell served as Lord Protector until his death in 1658 when the monarchy was restored under Charles II. The Church of England shored up its power under Charles II, with the establishment of the Clarendon code.[1]

All this was recent history when, in 1660, influenced by Francis Bacon's works, the Royal Society was founded, a learned gathering of the most illustrious scientists of Britain. In 1667 a member of the Society, Thomas Sprat, wrote a "History of the Royal Society" and dedicated it to King Charles II, as *de facto* head of the Church of England.[2] It is believed that Sprat was concerned that the persecution that scientists all over Europe were experiencing from the Catholic Church might spread to England and to the Church of England. He sought to safeguard the rights of British scientists by promising that scientists would "meddle no otherwise with divine things," and would limit their studies to the "constitution of the body" and the "works of their hands."[3] He further promised that scientists would not investigate "God and the soul."[4] Sprat's strategy appears to have been a success. Charles II was fond of the Royal Society, and every British monarch subsequent to Charles II has been a patron of the Society.

By this document, religious institutions, particularly the Church of England, were ceded the sole right to discuss and explore matters of the spirit, while scientists restricted themselves to exploration of material reality. Thus, in an unassuming fashion, from religious and political strife, scientific Materialism was born. Implicit in this artificial division was an attempt to placate both Catholic and Protestant theologians. The Earth, its people, and its material substance are granted to be something separate from Divinity, something less than Divine. A scientist could study God's handiwork, but not the mystery of the Divine itself or its connection with physical reality. This bargain was apparently acceptable to the Church, and Western science began to purposefully ignore the spiritual.

It has been largely forgotten that Materialism was a solution manufactured as a response to seventeenth-century English politics and religious tensions. Most people today have no idea that the separation of science and spirit was a bargain with the Church. Pretty much everyone in that era believed in God, and in a greater non-physical reality, whatever the nuances of their interpretation. Even the church of that era did not really believe in the separation, but it certainly wanted to be fully in charge of the peoples' understanding of spirit. Science could focus upon matters of the physical body only because the Church found the body less important than the soul. Particular doctrines about spirit were deemed so crucial that only ordained clergy could expound upon them.

Religion was very powerful in that era, and its leaders could not have foreseen that this seemingly small concession would be one of the major reasons for the downfall of its absolute control over the populace. The stage was set for the subsequent development of contemporary Western science, free of religious dogma and authority, but artificially divorced from any spiritual underpinnings or connection with a greater non-physical reality. The Church continues to expound upon non-physical reality, the afterlife, and eternity. But actual physical life, the life we know, is discussed only in the language of mechanistic science.

The birth of Materialism unfortunately has led to the contemporary belief that science and technology are separate from spirit, or that spirit simply does not exist because it has not been observed in scientific examinations. The time has come to mend this rift, because something cannot be observed if the very subject remains taboo. We will not observe anything that we are not, at the very least, open to observing. In Western scientific thought, we are trained to avoid seeing spirit. So it is not surprising that the spiritual only appears in the cracks. Science and spirit today are perceived as separate because they were separated for political and theological reasons. They remain separated because people no longer understand that any sort of unity exists. This has led to alienation in modern-day life, which also seems devoid of spirit.

The divided viewpoint has taken on a life of its own. There are many other ways of perceiving reality, even scientific reality. This can easily be seen in examining the majority of the traditions of the world in which there is no mind-body split, and no subsequent Materialism. While these diverse schools of thought reflect their own cultures, there is an implicit understanding in each of their philosophies and sciences of an underlying unity.

No mind-body split exists in traditional Asian philosophies. For example, in Buddhist thought, human beings are termed *Namarupa*, a Sanskrit conjugate of two terms: *Nama*, which means "name" and refers to the emotional and psychological attributes of a person, and *rupa*, which means "form" and refers to the physical structure of humans. These are combined into a single word and are thought to be unified, interdependent aspects of a person. They are neither separate nor separable.

In health sciences, there are many worldwide models of differing scientific viewpoints that developed without Materialism. Two well-known examples are Ayurveda and Traditional Chinese Medicine.

Ayurveda is the traditional healing system of India. This medical philosophy interweaves the physical and non-physical bodies into a seamless whole. A system of *chakras*, or non-physical energy centers, governs higher functioning of physical, emotional, and spiritual life. These energy centers are often depicted superimposed upon the physical body, but in Ayurvedic understanding they are a series of interconnected spinning spheres that contain the body. Ayurvedic medicine has a concept of a biofield, an energy field outside the physical body. In Ayurveda, the mind resides outside the body, and the higher mind is non-local, not fixed to any location.

Traditional Chinese Medicine, or TCM, also developed without a mind-body split. While the Chinese Communist regime of the twentieth century tried to expunge any purely spiritual references from the contemporary practice of TCM, they are found extensively in older Chinese medical texts. Since there was never, even in contemporary Communist TCM, a mind-body split, psychology in this system remains linked with physical health. Thus an illness like "liver invading spleen" might lead to digestive disturbance, irritability, menstrual problems in women, and feelings of frustration, while a kidney deficiency might include physical problems like urinary incontinence and frequent infections as well as emotional difficulties like fearfulness, timidity, and anxiety. In older Chinese texts, frankly spiritual material was interwoven into an understanding of the physical body. The entire journey of life is about the transformation of *jing*, or essence, into wisdom.

In an ironic twist of fate, the most spiritual tradition of Chinese medicine survives today exclusively in the West. Various scholars, especially the Jesuits, brought it out of China in the pre-Communist dynastic era. Today a spiritual understanding of human life and its relationship to the physical and emotional body remains central to certain types of Chinese medicine such as five-elements acupuncture.

There are many more examples of societies that understood the intertwining connection between physical and non-physical reality. It is fair to say, anthropologically, that almost all civilizations besides our current Western-dominated one understood that our world is encompassed by a greater non-physical reality. The advanced societies of ancient Egypt and the Incan and Mayan empires took spiritual reality literally and employed spiritual principles in every area of their science including medicine, architecture, technology, and design. Certainly no tribal peoples or civilizations had or have a mind-body split. Some, like the Aboriginal Australians, the Brazilian Yanomami, and the Bushmen of Southern Africa, had very little technology because of an utter reliance upon a relationship with the natural world. Others, like the natives of Southwestern U.S. who built the Canyon de Chelly monuments, and the ancient peoples of the Neolithic British Isles and Easter Island, built huge stone temples aligned with perfect precision to sophisticated astronomical coordinates. We still do not understand how they accomplished these feats. We do know that none of these cultures had a mind-body or soul-body split, and none were at war with nature or exhibited the destructive tendency of contemporary technology.

In the twentieth and twenty-first centuries, the mind-body dichotomy of Descartes has been rejected philosophically by many thinkers, but it persists in areas of the biological and medical sciences. But in diverse areas including neuroscience, quantum physics, humanistic psychology, sociobiology, and computer science, the understanding that there is an underlying unity of body and mind has largely replaced a mind-body dichotomy. There is no observable place, such as Descartes's pineal gland, where a division occurs. In many spiritual and scientific viewpoints, the physical body is an extension of thought. Body, mind, emotions, and spirit are inseparable, and an influence on one will affect all the others. This corresponds well to the observations of some contemporary quantum physicists who agree that there is no external material reality independent of the mind/consciousness that observes and influences it. This also dovetails well with such concepts as morphic resonance[5] and biofields that surround every living thing.

There are other ways of viewing reality. The seventeenth-century church did not want these to prevail, and many contemporary factions agree with that position. If people can communicate directly with spirit or with God, then religious institutions are not required as intermediaries. This might translate to a big loss of power for organized religions.

Mystics, however, often speak of the divine union that exists between humans and nature. Since early childhood, I can recall experiencing periods of union with the natural world. Trees talk to me in susurrations of the wind; birds fly overhead or call to me at just the right moment. The more I am in a relaxed state of well-being or joy, the more magical synchronicities weave through my day.

On the day I wrote this chapter, I took a walk in a nearby field, relaxing and contemplating what I wanted to say. Each time I had an insight that sparked me, small fluttering birds danced a confirmatory dance of delight in my line of sight. Each time I noted a complete concept on my digital voice recorder, a cluster of them flew directly overhead, or swooped playfully in front of me. Nature loves to engage us. She relishes childlike delight, silliness, and sheer joy and responds to these in kind. The ability to have mutually conscious joyful interaction with a living presence of nature is inherent in each of us.

Since my youth I have referred to the feeling of immanence in the natural world, the feeling of interacting with a living presence, as "the Green World." When I enter the Green World, all of nature is alive and humming. Sounds are clearer, the air is charged with visible light particles, and colors are intensely vivid. Everything seems to glisten, and the air is electric with a vibrant energy. In the Green World I understand myself as a part of nature, interconnected with all that I perceive. The usual beings of our world—plants, trees, rocks, soil, flowers, bacteria, and mycorrhizae—are present in the Green World, but everything is more vital and alive. I am easily able to connect with the life in the rocks or the wind when I am in the Green World.

I believe many children naturally step into the world of green when they have unstructured time in nature.

In my Green World interactions I may perceive messages. One day while I was working in my garden, considering where to place some new plants, I observed that the bees were not happy. (I am a bee-keeper and the bees live in my backyard.) They transmitted a thought that I interpreted as "We don't want to sting you but go away!" Three times bees came very close to my head, only my head, and the message was clearer each time. They meant business! The bees did not explain to me why they wanted me out of there. I had worked in my garden near them numerous times and felt a sense of peace from them. Perhaps perceiving that bees are giving a warning is not the Green World, but hearing their voice is. A few days later I was in the garden, not planting, and the bees were once again fine with my presence. About a week later I met with a permaculture consultant who nixed a lot of the plant choices I had made, including the very ones I had planned to plant the day the bees shooed me away. She helped me to choose a different selection of bee-friendly, long-blooming perennials better suited to my bioregion. The bees and I had cooperated on a preferable plan.

I also perceive what I refer to as "the Silver World." It is a symbolic world and is visible physically as well. In the Silver World, I find it easiest to communicate with the essences of things. I call it the Silver World simply because of its appearance when I was small; there is a silvery gleaming quality to the light. The Silver World is brighter and sparklier than the Green World. In the Silver World time is disjointed from ordinary flow. Events can be instantaneous, as in dreams, where one simply thinks of something and it materializes. Manifestations occur like the spark of an epiphany, while time has a slow, gelatinous flow. In the Silver World other beings are visible that are unseen in the normal world. There are gnomes and sprites and fairy-like creatures. The trees here sometimes have eyes, mouths, and hair. Normal physical objects might appear very different. A gnarl in a tree trunk can smile; eddies in water become water sprites that can giggle and dance and play with me. Colors are more vivid and rainbows glisten.

What is most important to me is the feeling of well-being I notice there. The Silver World is a joyous place where I always experience love. I also become suffused with energy and clarity that persists when I return to our normal world. I believe that many paranormal experiences are phenomena of the Silver World—miracles like a mother lifting a car off her trapped child, or a person in a bomb blast site seeing the whole situation in slow motion as she traverses a span out of harm's way that would be physically impossible, or people who report that beings of great light or their dead loved ones carried them out of burning buildings.

As a child, I thought these were actual places I was visiting, like fairy kingdoms. The terms Green World and Silver World were my personal referents from early childhood, and I found that I could get to the Silver World more easily by going through the Green World, like a doorway within a doorway. As an adult, I am now aware that both of these "places" are states of extraordinary perception. The Green World is a state of immanence, a state of attunement with nature in the moment. The Silver World is most like what has been described as the Devic realm or even a heavenly realm. It is a proverbial Garden of Eden in the mind's eye, or a Shambhala or an Avalon, and it is right there mixed in sidewise with the rest of physical reality. The Silver World is physical and is available here; though I now believe it may be a different dimension. Beings I perceive there are often archetypal. A single tree speaks for all trees, and a perfect rose for the essence of rosiness. I believe newborn babies live mostly in the Silver World, and many young children do too, or in the world of Green. That is why magic and fairy stories make so much sense to them. There is some science supporting this notion. The brain-wave patterns of a normal infant are identical to those of adept meditators in deep meditation.[6] Deep meditation, for adults, is one route to connection with expanded states of perception.

While writing this book I spent a great deal of time in the Silver World. I have been honored by visits from the Deva of Fleas and have been transported to the palace of rats, powerful experiences I discuss in a later chapter. In both worlds I frequently see lots of eyes. I believe this sighting is a playful cosmic joke. Many "eyes" all around is many "I's." Eyes are the I-others seeing me, as well as the eye-I me seeing aspects of myself.

There is also a Golden World, which I explored freely in early childhood and then lost conscious awareness of until I had a spontaneous mystical awakening experience at age nineteen. In the Golden World there is infinite light, or some vibration so high and pure it can only appear to a human mind's eye as golden light. This gold is not a color of the visible spectrum; it is a sensory light that requires no eyes to see. The light is all there is; it forms the basis of all things, physical and non-physical. In the Golden World I know everything, I connect with everything, and everything is perfection. Time does not exist here. It is not even relevant. There is a sound, a reverberation that encompasses all sound. The sound is serene, magnificent, infinitely complex, and simple all at the same time. It harbors all the beauty and majesty of sound yet is not audible to ears. It is audible, nonetheless, to consciousness. The light and sound of the Golden World are similar. There is a synesthesia of this world that I have never been able to accurately express. Light, sound, taste, and exultant feelings all intermingle. The Golden World fills and overflows all the senses.

My adult experience of the sensory fullness of the Golden World encompassed all paradox, dropping me in a place of unshakable inner peace that resides in my core. After this reconnection with the Golden World at age nineteen, my life course was profoundly altered. The feelings and perceptions have never fully left me, although they remain almost impossible to describe. I understood the meaning of "ineffable" after that experience. I understood that within and through me, and through each of us, is that which is ineffable. The experience of the Golden World is a being-ness, a wholeness, greater than physical existence. Others who have had similar encounters confirm that it leads to a radical shifting of perception that changes life thereafter.[7] The Golden World centers one firmly in the heart. It is a space of sustained knowing of grace beyond all illusions. It is the place, I believe, from which we are animated, from which our hearts beat in reverberation to the great heart of love creating us anew in every moment.

I now see that all of these worlds, and other nuanced layers, are superimposed upon our ordinary existence. The catch is that the texture is visible only to the allowing eye, tutored by the wise heart. The more I have allowed myself to step into the worlds of Green, Silver, and Gold, the more I see the magic that is all around us. It is spoken in the breeze, in the rustling of leaves and the crackling of a shower of berries landing on soil enriched by decaying leaves. It is also in the soil of my body, in the nuance of communication from my digestive tract to my larger consciousness.

I am not unique in my ability to see, nor is my ability to have these experiences unique. Everyone has the capacity to communicate with the natural world. We are all animated from the same eternal rhythm. It is inborn, an innate capacity as basic as the body's ability to heal, if we only get out of its way.

Currently a new paradigm is emerging (or, quite possibly, reemerging) on our planet. One way it is manifesting is that increasing numbers of individuals acknowledge their ability to communicate with a variety of beings. Some channel non-physical energies, some communicate telepathically with enlightened extraterrestrials, and others move between dimensions. Books are being written about communication with angels, dolphins, Pleiadeans, ascended masters, and God. People work as animal communicators and psychic healers. There is a burgeoning awakening and acceptance of our telepathic skills.

If more and more people find it easy to communicate with angels, non-physical beings, and extraterrestrials, it is understandably just as simple to communicate with the small, animate physical beings of our planet: insects, bacteria, protozoa, fungi, and viruses. Ultimately we learn that we can and do commune directly with life force itself as it moves through the greatest and the smallest. In fact, to life force, there is no great or small, there is only divine love.

I am confident that as more of us explore these experiences, we will coin new terms to describe them. One example of a recently minted term I love is "biophilia." It literally means a love of life or of living things, and its common usage implies a connection among all living things. "Philia" is in direct opposition to "phobia." Philia is an attraction toward another, while phobia is a fear of another. There is a biophilia hypothesis promulgated by biologist Edward O. Wilson, which says that we are genetically predisposed toward love of the natural world. I would go beyond this, understanding that love of nature is innate in us, not merely coded in our genes, but woven into every fiber of our being. We are nature. It is natural to love ourselves and it is natural to love the world around us.

We are creating new science that reflects this love. With our interwoven, interconnected planet it is now possible to link wisdom from traditional fields like Ayurveda and Chinese medicine to exciting research in quantum physics, parapsychology, astronomy, and health sciences. We can learn, for example, to work with a medicine of tone, color, light, and waveform that seems like magic or wish fulfillment today. Tomorrow there will be solid research to back it up. New science and new understanding are emerging everywhere, heralded by changes in physics that are spilling over into architecture, mathematics, engineering, and high tech. Lasers, holograms, and fractals are just a few of the early wave of practical applications available from the changes now upon us. As more of us understand that it is easy to move between the worlds, to see the bigger picture and to practically apply our broader comprehension, the creative blossoming will be even more magnificent than we can currently imagine.

Tools for Transformation

1. The system of chakras is one map of our physical energy-body world. It was developed in the Ayurvedic tradition of India. A simple technique that I have taught patients for many years is "chakra breathing." The chakras are energy centers of the emotional or spiritual body. The word "chakra" comes from the Hindu tradition, but these same energy centers have been observed in diverse other societies, including that of the Hopi. Catholic monks and mystics are also known to work with body-centered breathing techniques, especially those centering in the heart. If the idea of chakras seems foreign to you, imagine the different anatomical areas and the technique will work just as well.

   There are seven major chakras on and around the body, and many minor ones as well, but I am only mentioning a few of them here.

   The first exercise I give patients, especially if they are bothered by lots of thoughts, is to breathe in through the top of the head and out through the heart. Obviously anatomically we are breathing in through our nostrils or mouth and into our lungs, and out via the same orifices. But employing our imagination, we can see/feel our breath coming in through the top of our head and out through our heart/heart center located at the center of the breastbone (sternum). Doing so, we observe dynamic effects. This simple tool gets people out of the spinning thoughts of their head, and into the calm center of their heart. It also helps them to access universal wisdom by grounding it firmly in a heart-centered perspective. I have taught and practiced this simple technique since my early twenties, long before I was a physician, and find it immediately calming.

The flow of breath and energy can be reversed as well. Play with this. Breathe in through the heart and out through the top of the head. Notice what types of thoughts, feelings, sensations, and impressions are stimulated by each of these modes. This first exercise works with the crown chakra, where we connect to higher spiritual realms, the mind, where we receive thoughts and impressions, and the heart, the central chakra of the physical body and the seat of divine love.

2. To balance emotions, it is almost always soothing to practice breathing in through the heart and out through the gut. This can be any area of the abdomen that holds tension or discomfort. Many people report that their stomach gets knotted with tension when they are distressed. In those moments, they are not digesting the emotional content of their life experience. This type of breathing is calming and helps people connect their heart with their "gut feelings." Breathing between the heart chakra and the third chakra (or stomach area, just below the diaphragm) connects the heart with the emotional body, balancing both. In the chakra model, the third chakra (counting from the bottom up) is the location where emotions are processed in the spiritual body.

3. Breathing through the lower abdomen, about two inches below the navel, establishes a link with the second chakra. It is the seat of moving Qi and helps us feel connected to others and to the Earth. Breathing between the heart and the lower abdomen helps people to feel grounded, with a sense of belonging in the world.

So the next time you are tense, feel out of control, or experience any distress, try a few refreshing breaths, in through the heart, out through the stomach, or in through the heart, out through the lower abdomen. You may find, as have many of my patients, that this simple technique connects our "gut feelings" with the wisdom of the heart, allowing us to make better-feeling, more heart-centered choices and decisions, moment by moment, and day by day.

—CHAPTER EIGHT—

Balance

ALL BEINGS LIVE WITH ONE another in a state of dynamic and constantly changing balance. As one organism thrives, another declines. There is a perpetual recycling of the raw materials of life that make up our physical bodies. Minerals like carbon, calcium, magnesium, silica, and iron are the basic building blocks of life. All the minerals in our world today were created by the death of ancient stars incomprehensibly distant from us. We are alive because supernovae exploded and died in distant galaxies billions of years ago, spewing the dust that is now our flesh across the chasm of space. We are stardust.

While alive, each organism strives to promote the conditions that enhance its own survival and the survival of its offspring. Classical Darwinism frames this self-interest in terms of competition for scarce resources, but collaboration for mutual benefit is more commonly the result. Frequently there is interspecies cooperation occurring of which neither is fully conscious. For example, for most of human civilization, we did not give any thought to our intestinal bacteria because we did not even know they were there. The bacteria probably do not think of us consciously either, certainly not in the way humans do. But for hundreds of thousands of years, bacteria existed inside of us, living their lives. Their flourishing was synonymous with our flourishing.

Enhancement of survival can occasionally result in competition for territory, but the classical warlike interpretation of Darwin's work is being replaced by a more expansive recognition of the central importance of collaboration. Even Darwin modified and softened his understanding in his later works, placing much more emphasis on relationship and partnership as forces that shape evolutionary change. In his second pivotal work, *The Descent of Man*, Darwin writes of the evolutionary advantage of mutual cooperation, especially within species. He implies that within a species, the fittest are those that co-operate the best. He wrote: "Those communities which included the greatest number of the most sympathetic members would flourish best, and rear the greatest number of offspring."[1]

A modern writer, David Loye, expounds on Darwin's observations in his books, *Darwin's Lost Theory of Love* (2000) and the revised version *Darwin's Lost Theory* (2007). He believes that Darwin has been misunderstood and misrepresented. Loye maintains that Darwin's greatest contribution was an understanding that human evolution is dependent upon our moral capacity, compassion, and a desire for the good of others, rather than selfishness or mere self-preservation. Amity, mutuality, and rapport enhance survival within the human species.

So I am not the first to consider the advantages of a model of co-operation in the evolutionary process. Despite the Darwinism that children continue to be taught in schools, over the last forty or so years there has been a quiet revolution in our understanding of evolution. In a September 2005 article in the journal *Common Ground*, Geoff Olson revisited a 1991 essay titled "Kropotkin Was No Crank" by Harvard paleontologist Stephen Jay Gould. Both articles examine the life and work of the Russian geographer Alexeivich Kropotkin. In his youth, Kropotkin was deeply enamored by Darwin's ideas, but as an officer and a geographer in Siberia he observed much greater evidence for cooperation enhancing survival, especially among members of the same species. In 1902 Kropotkin authored a book titled *Mutual Aid: A Factor in Evolution.*

Olson makes a number of important points, and the entire article is worth reading. He points out:

> The evidence supporting Kropotkin's thesis is now substantial. The many examples of mutualism and symbiosis are too numerous to touch on here, other than a few prominent

examples from the very beginnings of life. Among the first species of bacteria, it is now believed, three organisms lived in cozy symbiosis as the cooperative precursors to animal cells' organelles—the nucleus, mitochondria, and centrioles. Another variety of cell began to live in association with organisms capable of photosynthesis, in turn evolving into plant cells with their light-munching chloroplasts. This kind of micro-cooperation persists to this day ... Without a substantial level of collaboration between and within species, from the micro to the macro, life would not likely have evolved much past simple self-replicating strands of DNA.[2]

New research on bacteria demonstrates that "both the fit and the unfit coexist indefinitely," thus enhancing diversity.[3] It turns out that cooperative relationships are more frequently the norm than competitive ones. Survival of the fittest usually means something more akin to "plays nicely with others." Instinctively, this makes sense. It seems reasonable that peaceful mutualism enhances survival more than continual competition and fighting. Human fighting and wars consume lives and fracture communities. Peaceful, tranquil times create eras of abundance.

It is logical that other species also flourish best during times of peace. Climax forest ecosystems thrive when multiple species find balance, and decline after clearcuts and "managed forest plantations" of tree monocultures (the forest equivalent of war) replace them. Bee colonies multiply when they remain in one location, when there are diverse species of flowering plants to provide them nectar and honey, and in the absence of chemical pesticides and herbicides (their equivalent of war).

"Resilience" is a term now utilized to describe complex interactive systems. There are large databases on resilience that examine its applicability in diverse arenas including human psychology, governments, engineering, political structures, and wetlands. The concept is used to understand individuals, families, communities, cultures, financial institutions, and ecosystems. Resilience provides a model for understanding the variety of factors that may impinge upon a complex system and its adaptive capacity. Resilience theory acknowledges that the whole is greater than the sum of its parts. A fabric of many relationships, taken as a whole, determines whether a system will collapse with disturbance, shift to a new stable state, or be restored.

Our complexity forces us to find ways to look at life as a web of relationships. In holistic medicine, the emerging concept of biological terrain reflects an understanding of the body as an interrelated web of organisms. It is one example of a model for understanding health and disease that differs from the currently widespread biomedical paradigm. According to biological terrain, each of us is a whole world, comprised of many smaller ecosystems and niches. As a society, we are a community of worlds.

As I mentioned in an earlier chapter, the human body is comprised of many terrains: sinuses are marsh-like, exposed skin is arid, and skin creases and folds are more damp and moist, much like soil. Ideal conditions for various functions or symbioses arise in each environment. Healthy skin is slightly acidic while blood is slightly alkaline. We are a host for trillions of organisms, some of which, like little "Whos in Whoville," themselves host a multitude of organisms. Microbes that are commonplace and benign in one region of the body, like *Staph aureus* on skin, can cause disease in other areas, like the eye or gastrointestinal tract.

All these organisms in and on us want the same thing—survival and thriving of their own. They do not think about this like you or I do, but they have an instinctual imperative to flourish as best they can. Organisms help create environments that support their own flourishing and the well-being of their offspring. Thus fungus will create a more alkaline pH in mucous membranes such as the vagina or the colon, while bacteria we consider "healthy" for our immune systems, such as *Lactobacillus acidophilus* and *bifidus*, prefer a slightly acidic pH in these same membranes.

These concepts matter for our health. We feel uncomfortable when conditions favorable to yeast growth predominate in our body, and we feel more vitality when the "normal flora" flourish. The concept of biological terrain has been a dominant undercurrent in medicine for more than one hundred years. In the late 1800s, there was a rivalry between two brilliant scientists: Louis Pasteur and Claude Bernard. Bernard favored the concept of biological terrain, stating that "the host is everything and the organism is nothing." What he meant by this is that resilience is determined by the overall state of health and well-being of the host individual, and not the virulence of particular pathogenic organisms. Pasteur, during much of his lifetime, studied the virulence of microorganisms, but it is said (perhaps as an urban legend) that near the end of his life he conceded that Bernard's view was the more correct one. Unfortunately, most scientists to this day still operate from Pasteur's limited model and few have heard of Claude Bernard.

Much of what we now think of as "modern" medicine is an outgrowth of the earlier, incomplete understanding of Pasteur, combined with the warlike competitiveness of classical Darwinism. We have gone far down this path and now appear to be nearing the end of it, simply because it is too reductionistic. It is obvious that the virulence of an organism or a disease is not the only factor in health or illness. Some people exposed to the flu will not get sick; others will be ill for weeks. Some people who contract Lyme disease are asymptomatic, others are desperately ill. For almost every organism there is a range of responses in human beings from no symptoms or a few mild symptoms to serious or perhaps life-threatening illness. People can even sicken from infections of normal flora overgrowth.

I wondered why, for example, are there so many asymptomatic carriers of illnesses like Lyme disease and a few desperately ill ones?

The very existence of this paradoxical situation makes the whole field of Lyme treatment controversial. The conventional model addresses Lyme disease as a short-term illness to be treated by three to four weeks of antibiotics. On the other hand, there are some critically ill persons who seemingly exhibit years of intractable and disabling Lyme.

Even diagnosis is tricky. The Centers for Disease Control (the CDC) has one set of rigorous criteria for establishing who has Lyme. Under their strict standards, few people actually qualify for this booby prize. New York state, a hotbed of Lyme cases, where even the CDC admits there are four to five times as many cases as in other locations, has a slightly more expanded but similar set of criteria to the CDC. Lyme specialist physicians, conversely, have entirely different and much broader standards for determining who is affected. There is so much back and forth arguing about this that it is difficult to say how many people have been affected. Officially the number of cases in the United States is about eight persons per 100,000, but people in the Lyme community surmise that the actual prevalence of infection might be exponentially higher.

For me, Lyme has become a symbol for the canon of belief in solely external causation of illness. I work with a number of patients with Lyme disease, some of whom meet the CDC criteria and others who do not. All measure up to some yardstick for determination of Lyme cases. While I acknowledge that certain patients are quite ill, I do not believe this is solely due to a tiny corkscrew-shaped bacteria. The presence of Lyme spirochetes is only one factor that determines health or illness. Other pivotal factors include underlying health and immune status, toxic burden, general well-being and happiness, gastrointestinal health or lack of it, constitutional factors including genetics, and acute and ongoing stressors.

In my experience, the Lyme patients who have made the most progress have let go of the attachment to merely blaming a bacterial

organism for their problems and have begun to look more expansive-
ly at many factors, including questions of meaning, joy, and well-being
in their lives. They have stopped focusing exclusively on killing (and
hating) the Lyme and have instead devoted themselves to improving
their overall health and well-being in many areas of their lives. Not
all of them do this. For some people, illness has become their identity.
These people are typically fearful and quite attached to their image
of themselves as sick. I do not try to persuade them otherwise. When
a patient believes there is no hope for recovery, there probably isn't
any. For them, I merely try to give ease where I can. If patients latch
on to words of hope, I will pick up that ball and move forward with
it along with them. But if they argue against hope, I will simply offer
comfort and continue to treat them as best I can.

One patient, "Lawrence," in his mid fifties, struggled with chronic
Lyme disease. Lyme had incapacitated him, though he still scrambled
to hang on to his ability to work twenty hours per week in order to
afford medications and his complementary therapy treatments. When
he first consulted me, he had a recent diagnosis of early prostate cancer as well. At that first visit he was joylessly plodding though life.
He had few friends, felt lonely and isolated, and worked at a job he
disliked. The small amount of work he did provided all the contact
he had with others.

How did he get here? Well, he had a very stressful divorce in
his early thirties, which is, not surprisingly, when he feels his health
problems began. He suspects he contracted the Lyme disease during
this period. He was also financially stressed at the time. He had been
"struggling" as a musician, but after marrying he gave this up and took
a job in computer programming. Lawrence never enjoyed this work;
in fact, he can list the many ways that he finds the job objection-
able. He remarked: "Its sole saving grace is that it pays well." He still
yearned for the freedom and promise of his younger years when he
planned a career in music and believed in his dreams. He sensed that

his life had "gone sour" and blamed illness and his divorce for his lack of verve.

We are taught self-doubt early in our lives, "for our own good." I very often see bright, talented young people, especially those who enjoy the arts and music, who are discouraged from pursuing their dreams. They slot themselves into careers with which they have no heart connection, often on the advice of others who have already given up their own dreams. Unless people find meaning in their new path, they set themselves up for an unsatisfying life. Beyond basic levels of sustenance, wealth does not increase happiness or quality of life.

Lawrence's situation reminds me of one of my favorite quotes from the Dalai Lama. When asked what surprised him most about humanity, the Dalai Lama answered, "Man.... Because he sacrifices his health in order to make money. Then he sacrifices money to recuperate his health. And then he is so anxious about the future that he does not enjoy the present; the result being that he does not live in the present or the future; he lives as if he is never going to die, and then dies having never really lived."[4]

Lawrence's ambivalence and regret lodged in his body, which promptly and cooperatively reflected this to him. The obliging Lyme organisms assisted in reminding him that he had veered from his chosen path. But he did not understand the message of the Lyme. He focused instead on his difficulties, sinking into despair and self-pity, and his problems compounded over many years. Eventually this all began to "eat away at him" and he developed cancer as well. Like most people, Lawrence did not understand that there was meaning to his illness. He believed things "just happen to us" and that he had "bad luck." When he consulted me, more than twenty years later, we delicately revisited the original question of the loss of meaning in his life and how it might be related to his various illnesses—not as a source of blame but as an opportunity for growth in the present.

Remarkably, Lawrence was ready for a turning point. He had already begun to wonder if there might be a different way to look at his circumstances. He began to play some music, at first just in his home, merely "fooling around." This reconnection with his passion gave him a lot of joy and helped him pleasantly pass the time during his cancer treatments. While he realized that the dreams of his youth were no longer viable in the same form as when he left them, he was able to rediscover his heart. He left the dead end of his old computer-programming job. Augmented by a little money "serendipitously" inherited from his parents, he took a training-wage position that involved more interesting (to him) facets of computer technology, as it dovetailed with music. He was quickly promoted twice in an eighteen-month period and now earns an hourly wage just below the amount he was earning when he left the job he deplored. He is optimistic about the future and enjoys his new line of work immensely. He enjoys going to work, loves its challenges, and admires the creativity of his co-workers. Lawrence is now able to work thirty hours per week without fatigue, while he used to drag through twenty. Most importantly, he understands that his happiness and satisfaction are essential for his health. Today his cancer is in remission and the Lyme is quite a bit less active, even though the only new treatment for the Lyme was letting go of the enmity with the organism and finding a way to love his life. He now smiles a lot and needs a lot less money for treatment, because he is significantly less ill.

There are many such stories, for there is a lot more going on than simple biochemistry. Health relates to the entirety of who we are. In contemporary medicine we like to believe that *a* causes *b* and results in *c,* but there is so much more complexity and variability in living systems that this is demonstrably not true. In modern industrial medicine, we are seeing the breakdown of reductionism. We are not little machines and we are not simply a mix of chemicals or amino acids. The very act of attempting to reduce living systems to isolated causes and effects guarantees that there are always more questions than answers. The body is not a simple mathematical equation or test-tube chemical reaction. We cannot input this and tidily get that.

What medical science does very well, in this increasing compartmentalization, is describe pathology. In medical texts and research reports, we find artful and detailed descriptions of what is occurring physiologically in illness. We can describe what some pharmaceuticals are doing and what is occurring in the body's processes. All of this is delivered with many descriptive long words and Latin phrases. There is no deep understanding of causation or relationship. For example, any diagnosis that ends with "itis" just means inflammation of that thing. So bronchitis is inflammation of the bronchi, while neuritis is inflammation of the nerves, and gastritis is inflammation of the stomach. Some "itises" are quite specific. Perioral dermatitis, for example, is inflammation of the area around the mouth. Absorbed in the eloquence of the descriptive language about *what* is occurring, it is easy to overlook that we have no clue about *why* these abnormal processes are happening.

Most pharmaceuticals merely block or stop some normal process of the body. They do this to affect symptoms, not causes. They are described by their actions, *what* they do, not *why* we have the problem in the first place. H2 blockers, a class of stomach acid production suppressants, stop histamine production, while statin drugs inhibit an enzyme called HMG co-A reductase that the liver uses to make cholesterol. There are huge gaps in our knowledge. Basic questions remain hanging. Are people who have heartburn really producing too much acid? You would think we know this for sure, but we do not. Some practitioners think that people with heartburn actually produce too little stomach acid. There is quite a bit of logic to this opinion. The pyloric valve at the far end of the stomach is the aperture through which partially digested food passes on to the intestines. Its opening is triggered by a sufficiently low stomach pH. When there is not enough stomach acid, food can churn and churn and eventually back up into the esophagus.

There are bigger questions as well. Why, all of a sudden in our society, are huge numbers of people having this problem? Is diet really irrelevant? Why does the liver make cholesterol? Isn't it found in every cell of our body?

Almost all the processes that are blocked by various drugs are normal, healthy processes. All are necessary for maintaining and restoring balance. What happens when we blockade normal physiologic processes in large swaths of the population? Does this constitute a cure? In the case of common heartburn, various antacids, acid suppressors, and acid blockers are commonly sold. Medicine does not ask why so many people have heartburn or reflux esophagitis today. It just describes what it believes is going on, and prescribes a drug to eliminate the symptom temporarily. Cute animated television commercials advertising illness promote the same limited ideology: "Take a pill, relieve the symptom!" Since nothing underlying changes, the patient finds herself endlessly on medication.

I have many patients, including Nan and Judith, with chronic reflux. Nan has been seeing a gastroenterologist and has been diagnosed with Barrett's esophagitis, a precancerous condition of the esophagus caused by chronic heartburn. She takes acid blockers every day and does not feel good about this, but she has felt unable to modify anything about her diet or her high stress level. She likes the refined flour and fried foods she is used to, and constantly worries about money; but she feels overwhelmed and powerless to make any changes. Nan eats as cheaply as possible, buying sale foods and bulk items from large commercial chains. Five years into her acid blockade program, Nan has developed two other problems. She now has fatty liver infiltration with abnormal liver tests, and severe gas and bloating. Her esophagus is no worse, it is true, but it is no better either. We both agree that the supplements I can offer her are not doing a lot of good.

Judith, on the other hand, was unwilling to settle for the diagnosis of chronic gastroesophageal reflux disease (otherwise known as GERD). She asked lots of questions about the balance of factors that could lead to this situation and had a strong desire to change them. She was willing to make significant adjustments in lowering her stress and digesting her life experience. She recognized that there are lots of tasty foods, and she could happily choose ones her body preferred. She accepted the premise that if her body asked for a different way of eating, she would honor herself by listening to it. She took stock of what she valued most about life and began to prioritize the things that were important to her, such as play-dates with her nieces and nephews, time in nature, and conversations with friends. She stopped watching the news at mealtimes and now listens to relaxing music or dines with a loved one.

Judith made a lot of changes, and in just two months she no longer needed acid blockers or antacids because she no longer ever had heartburn. After six months she had lost thirty excess pounds that had accumulated on her frame during her forties. She did not diet. Instead she paid attention to her body. She looked at the symptoms as an indicator of imbalances that she felt empowered to address.

The pretense of being able to control or micromanage physical manifestations that are ever more artfully described yet not really understood is one of the great failings of our current medical model. With all the glitz of medicine, doctors can actually permanently cure very few things. We cannot cure a common cold, gastroenteritis, or arthritis. Modern medicine is not geared toward curing; it is now mostly a system of disease management. Even curable illnesses, like type 2 diabetes and reflux esophagitis, are managed because we have a medical system that manages disease rather than addressing what is at the root of a problem.

Modern medicine developed as a system attached to no deeper moorings. There is no understanding of who we really are and what we are really doing here, so illness seems meaningless and random. This is not to say that doctors themselves are callous. Far from it. Most people who become physicians, nurses, and other health professionals genuinely care about others. They want to help. It is the medical system itself, based on flawed premises, that is inherently impaired.

Disease can be seen as shifting the balance in the biological terrain rather than as a tragedy. "Homeostasis" is a term that refers to self-maintaining balance in organisms. When our homeostasis is disturbed we exhibit signs of illness in an effort to restore balance. Dis-ease is a message from one's body about imbalance. When we "run ourselves ragged" over a short time, we may get a cold or flu as the body's way of quickly slowing us down. If we are healthy, we rebound rapidly. If we eat food that is spoiled and we are very healthy, we might vomit it up a short while later with no repercussions. In the model of resilience theory, these are imbalances the system can correct. The brief illness is the correction, restoring the system to its prior level of function.

If, over a long period of time, we eat foods that are devitalized, such as processed foods and "fast foods," because we are rushing through our lives without taking time to digest our experience or listen to our bodies and to actually prepare healthy foods at home, we may develop numerous gastrointestinal and degenerative problems that reflect our lack of physical and emotional nutrition. When we run our lives "on fumes" for long stretches, pushing ourselves through unhappiness day after day, through force of will, we may eventually get fatigue that can become chronic. The body tries to bring us back into balance by slowing us down more definitively. If we look at this through resilience theory we see that now the body of the ill individual has rebalanced in a newly reorganized adaptive state. This is not as ideal a state as the prior level of function. But because of the digestive problems, fewer damaging foods are offered since they are simply and clearly not tolerated; and because of the fatigue the person can no longer run himself or herself into the ground at the same pace. A new homeostasis was achieved at a cost. The body cuts its losses and moves on. Health is not vigorous, but function can continue. Finally, there are severe imbalances, like massive trauma, so great that the system cannot regain homeostasis. As a result of these the individual, like any ecosystem, perishes.

In Bernard's terms our individual ecosystem and terrain are the source of the imbalance. The biologic terrain model encompasses the interrelated nature of our "isolated" body systems, as well as the relationship between our physical body and the larger environment. Biological terrain acknowledges that it is difficult to have a healthy body in a severely ailing physical environment. Survivors of Chernobyl or Nagasaki suffered many sicknesses, physical and emotional.

The physical body is one unit. The endocrine system is intimately connected with the nervous system and the circulatory system. All of these affect the gastrointestinal tract. The health of the brain, including cognitive function, is intimately connected to the vitality of the gastrointestinal tract as well. The health of the heart relates to the health of the muscles. But modern medicine picks us apart into lots of tiny turfs. The endocrinologist works with the hormones, the cardiologist with the heart, and the pulmonologist with the lungs, as if these systems are not interrelated. Sick people acquire a collection of medical sub-specialists at cross-purposes who may not communicate with one another. We are definitely not a collection of unrelated organs and systems. Everything interacts and it's all intricately connected. Human health is about balance and relationship.

In the weird world of contemporary medicine, the more specialized a practitioner is, the higher the status and the higher the paycheck. Lowest paid, and least valued, are practitioners trying to grasp the bigger picture by looking at the whole person. You end up with a great deal of absurdity in such a system including gastroenterologists who claim it does not matter what a person eats, and cardiologists who commonly prescribe medicines that deplete nutrients essential for the heart—medicines that may ultimately cause new cases of heart disease. Industrialized medicine, I believe, has lost its understanding of health.

An unfortunately common scenario is the one I encountered with a new patient, Don. A formerly healthy and unmedicated sixty-five-year-old, Don visited a cardiologist on the advice of his family physician. Prior to this, Don was not ill. He was a non-smoker and teetotaler who exercised daily. He had never had a cardiac problem, but his father, a chain-smoking alcoholic, died of a heart attack at sixty-nine years old. Don had mildly "elevated" cholesterol levels, by the cardiologist's standards, so the cardiologist put him on a cholesterol-lowering medication. This medication caused severe chronic gout, and Don was unable to exercise as he previously had and gained twenty pounds. He consulted a rheumatologist regarding the gout, who put him on non-steroidal anti-inflammatory drugs for the pain and inflammation. After a few months on these medications, Don developed chronic gastritis. So he saw a gastroenterologist who put him on acid blockers for reflux. It was at this point that I met Don, after his daughter—already one of my patients—encouraged him to see someone who could look at the whole picture from a fresh perspective.

At our interview, I found Don to be affable and intelligent. He had silently questioned the wisdom of the first medication because he felt fine, but he said, "You hear so much these days about cholesterol, I was worried when my doctor told me I had it." He was surprised when I explained that everyone "has cholesterol," that it is in every cell of the body, and that looking at his levels, I saw that his were not even particularly high. Many doctors, myself included, would not consider medication in his situation. Don had not understood that the entire progression of illnesses was a line of dominoes falling down as his body repeatedly attempted to rebalance. Natural process after natural process was thwarted by further pharmaceutical interventions that were a direct result of side effects of the first medication. After discussing how all of these problems were interrelated and his range of choices, Don chose to go off the cholesterol-lowering medication causing the gout, as well as the anti-inflammatory. I suggested a four-week rebalancing diet and health program. One week into it, and off the other two medicines, Don tentatively went off the acid blocker as well. He was relieved to notice no heartburn. Four weeks later he was starting to feel like himself again, instead of "like an old man with one foot in the grave."

It is easy to see that by applying a system of resilience—one that understands that health is about balance—we get a lot more meaningful information. We can be empowered to recreate our vitality. We can eat nutrient-dense foods that help the normal flora of our body to thrive and will support our organs, skeleton, and endocrine system. Usually this means food that is fresh and local so that nutrients have not decayed. Also important is eating food free of pesticides, toxins, antibiotics, radiation, and hormones, and discontinuing use of products such as chemical-laden "room deodorizers" to minimize the challenge and stress on our bodies' detoxification capacity. We can move and stretch to support the normal flow of lymph by any number of fun exercises including walking, hiking, swimming, gardening, or yoga. This is ideal when we have a clean and safe environment in which to move about. We can find balance in our lives by choosing meaningful work, fulfilling hobbies, and harmonious relationships. Usually this means that we accept and believe in ourselves and know that we deserve happiness. Usually this also means that we have friends, family, and communities. All of these systems are intimately interrelated with our physical and emotional health.

All this matters greatly, and there is still a bigger picture. All illness begins in the realm of energy disruption. Specifically, illness begins with disruption of the smooth communication of our soul's purpose into our physical vehicle. All healing begins in the realm of energy rebalancing. If we are eternal beings whose purpose is joy, and if we are all related, then healing occurs in relationship to our soul. Meaning, purpose, compassion, creativity, and love are all essential elements in a healthy life lived in a thriving body.

TOOLS FOR TRANSFORMATION

1. Problem-solving meditations are a great tool for smoothly navigating life stressors and day-to-day decisions. Decision-making can be easier when we include the heart's wisdom and our intuitive capacity. There are many fun ways to engage our inner being at these levels. You can apply these tools when making decisions about health or health care, or any question you have.

   I always advise beginning any problem-solving session by centering. This can be accomplished by doing any of the heart-centered breathing exercises discussed in this book. You can also center by many other techniques. Walking meditations, such as walking a labyrinth, are fine ways to connect with your inner wisdom and calm. There are also many excellent guided meditations available as recordings or videos. Try a number of tools and see which one is best for you.

2. After you have centered and attained a feeling of calm, see your choices spread out before you as if they are different roads or paths through a wood. Peer down each of the roads and see which has more light. See which is more inviting, feels happier, and appears more interesting. I always encourage people to add another road or path than the ones they are aware of. For example, you may be deciding between whether to try a new medication that is being suggested for a current condition or a surgical procedure. If you put the medication on path "A" and the surgery on path "B," include a path "C" that is more vague—label it "some other choice." If it turns out that "C" clearly or even somewhat feels like the most attractive option, you will have some more research to do after your meditation.

3. Another problem-solving tool is to ask the question, then relax and center. When you are calm, imagine that your mind is a screen where a movie is about to start. Let go of asking the question and just watch the images that come up in response to it. See if they give you any insight.

4. When you are done, check in with your heart. Does your decision feel comfortable there? Do you feel resolved? A good decision should give you a feeling of peace and well-being.

—CHAPTER NINE—

Trust: Viruses

Trust can be a hard sell because it brings us to the heart of the self/other paradox. In a culture of fear, we are taught that we must control others for our own security and well-being, since they are unpredictable. The need for learning trust arises with the dawning realization that it is impossible to control external conditions in enough ways to ensure one's own happiness or comfort. Even a little bit of control of others requires excessive time and effort. Mostly, we can neither predict nor control the actions of others.

What do we actually control? Not our children, our parents, our spouses or lovers, or even our pets. Not the political arena, not the microbes in our bodies. Not corporations or the traffic on the roads we drive upon. Not "wild animals." We certainly do not control people who believe differently than we do and who have chosen dissimilar lifestyles. When we feel the need to control others for our own well-being, we are left with a feeling of powerlessness—due mainly to the false underlying premises of our culture. We believe we are at war. We are offered the false choice of trying to master the outcome of our personal experience by controlling "others." This includes individuals, aspects of the natural world, and even one's own body. The alternate choice we are offered culturally is passively accepting our circumstances without alteration. This is a false dichotomy.

Trust dawns in understanding that we do not need others to change for our well-being. Happiness, peace, and serenity are all an inside job. Trust implies letting go of our illusions of control. In actuality, we already do control everything essential to our well-being. We can control our thoughts, and we can control what we focus upon and how we think about it. No one else can make us think about something. No one can force our attention to any topic, though we may have habits so ingrained that it feels, especially initially, that we are compelled. We may believe that our limited-state perception is normal, reinforcing it by repeating adages like "You can't teach an old dog new tricks."

But we can shift. Amusingly, trainer Cesar Millan has shown us in his program that even very old dogs can learn new tricks. My dog Lily used to strain at the leash and bark aggressively every time we passed another dog on the sidewalk. Trainers we consulted in the past told us there was nothing we could do about this unpleasant situation. So for years we avoided walking near other dogs while Lily was on a leash, criss-crossing the street when needed. She is an old dog, eleven to be exact, and it took only one weekend of applying tools from Millan's program to shift this supposedly deeply ingrained, "unchangeable" behavior. Lily is now a pleasurable companion on or off leash.

At any age, and despite any prior conditioning, we humans can transform our lives by working with thoughts, beliefs, focus, and ourselves. We can give greater value to joy, love, and happiness. Our basic physiology indicates that essential functions including cellular repair, hormone balance, and immune activity are all dependent upon emotional well-being and self-love for optimal activity. For example, one of the keys to proper immune function is the production of endogenous opiates. In plain English, this means that each of us manufactures natural opiates, called endorphins. People who have higher levels of these hormones of well-being enjoy better moods than those who do not. We can increase our endorphin production by increasing exercise as well as retraining our thoughts to focus more positively. Our physical and emotional health can thrive as we develop new habits.

The current medical model sees the body as nature, something to be conquered. Trying to subdue the wildness within us, medicine perpetuates a misunderstanding, so any underlying chances of real resolution go out the window. Our alignment with our inner self—as expressed in our level of peace, joy, and serenity—is an essential factor in health and illness. Real healing lies in recognizing and tuning harmoniously to the voice of our soul, thereby creating harmony and coherence in our bio-energetic field.

Medically, the issue of fear and control versus trust and love is epitomized by our relationship with viruses. In this arena there is an inherent lack of trust. There is so much we do not know about viruses. Perhaps this wariness is partly because the word "virus" is derived from a Latin root meaning "toxin," "venom," or "poison." We clearly were not expecting or planning an amicable relationship from the moment viruses were discovered. *Merriam-Webster's Dictionary Online* defines "virus" this way:

1. *archaic:* venom
2a. the causative agent of an infectious disease
  b. any of a large group of submicroscopic infective agents that are regarded either as extremely simple microorganisms or as extremely complex molecules, that typically contain a protein coat surrounding an RNA or DNA core of genetic material but no semi-permeable membrane, that are capable of growth and multiplication only in living cells, and that cause various important diseases in humans, lower animals, or plants; *also:* filterable virus
  c. a disease or illness caused by a virus
3. something that poisons the mind or soul <the force of this *virus* of prejudice—V. S. Waters>
4. a computer program that is usually hidden within another seemingly innocuous program and that produces copies of itself and inserts them into other programs and usually performs a malicious action (as destroying data).[1]

After reading these definitions, I would add to our current conception of virus the words "sneaky" and "intentionally malicious." There has been debate since the first virus was discovered as to whether these are "anima," i.e., whether they are life forms or not. They have some properties we recognize in life: they have genes (DNA or RNA) and they reproduce. In reproducing they consume nutrients, and they can evolve and change. However, they do not have a cell wall or other aspects of cellular structure. Only a lipid or protein coat covers viruses. They live within host cells and utilize the host cells' metabolic machinery. They do not exhibit cell division. Instead, viruses assemble inside host cells and are released, sometimes gradually and sometimes exuberantly, when they rupture the cell, leading to the cell's death. Viruses do not exhibit biological activity outside host cells.

There is much more unknown about viruses than known. We have no idea how viruses originated. Did they evolve along with other life forms? Are they an example of devolution—parasitic life forms that once were independent and now are dependent on host cells? Could viruses be an intermediate or proto-life form? In the 1950s a group of three scientists demonstrated that tobacco mosaic virus would form spontaneously when its genomic RNA was incubated with a purified protein coat. But this finding has not been reproduced with other types of viruses. Are they new life forms? All of these are theories currently in fashion. Then there are more outlandish possibilities, equally plausible, including the theory that viruses originated in space, or in our minds, that they have group intelligence like bees, or that they are organelles of a larger consciousness.

What if most viruses were not harmful, in most circumstances? What if they were helpful? What if, as is the case, our bodies harbor billions of viruses at any given time that exhibit no pathological activity? Although we have no clue what they are doing, they might have important physiologic functions in our homeostasis (self-regulation). Perhaps, like bacteria, there are beneficial activities of viruses for human, plant, and animal health. What if viruses were not sneaky interlopers, out to harm, but just tiny proto-organisms on their own life trajectories? What if they are proto-organisms that intersect with our trajectories based upon our vibrations and not upon their will or malice? What if that viral life trajectory intersects with other living species, sometimes beneficially, sometimes neutrally, and occasionally with apparent detriment?

Virologists recognize that viruses can enter cells and remain dormant for extended periods of time, during which the host cells do not appear to be changed. This is known as a lysogenic phase. When viruses become activated or stimulated, they enter a reproductive phase, called the lytic phase, where new virus particles assemble in the cell and eventually rupture it, resulting in the release of the particles. There are also virus particles that can enter a cell but are unable to reproduce.

There are ways in which viral infections enhance our immune system. When we get the common cold, it is an opportunity for our body to clean out old toxins and metabolic wastes. People who get periodic colds (once or twice a year) may be protected from more severe illnesses, like cancer, as they age.

We do not really know whether there are benefits from having dormant viruses in our system. I suspect there are, especially in the area of terrain modification. Just as we live harmoniously and symbiotically with beneficial bacteria, I believe it is likely we will discover the same is true of viruses. Many are likely to be protective, colonizing cells so potentially more dangerous organisms cannot thrive.

What about the virulence of viruses? Many viruses are not particularly infective. For example, among the picornaviruses, which include the polio virus, only one in a thousand particles is actually infective. Virologists consider the lack of virulence in viruses quite a challenge, as they must make many cultures to study an infection. However, as I assume nature does not make big mistakes, there must be an adaptive advantage to viruses that are non-virulent.

Our entire relationship with viruses is an arena where I believe much fruitful exploration, with the eyes of love, is waiting to emerge.

For example, viruses enter cells by attaching proteins, called "anti-receptors" to glycoprotein receptors on the cell surface. Attachment to the receptor sometimes permanently alters the virus, although in most cases, a virus can detach from a cell if it is not able to enter it. Viruses recognize which cells to enter by the presence of specific receptors on the cell surface. Let me say that again, because it is key. Specific receptors, already on the cell, indicate to viruses which cell is receptive to penetration and colonization. This implies that the cell itself, by exhibiting the presence of virus-specific receptors, has a vital role in choosing to be inhabited by a virus. There are similarities here with how the ovum very actively chooses the sperm that it will allow to enter. Like an egg being fertilized, once a virus attaches to a receptive cell, there is penetration.

After penetration a process called "uncoating" takes place. It is this phase that allows the virus to express its genome. How this happens is poorly understood. But often the host cell plays a part in whether or not the virus will express itself and replicate! It appears likely that we, or some aspect of ourselves, decide whether a virus living in us will express itself. Of course, this is not a conscious decision. People do not say to themselves, "I think I'll get a cold or flu now, or perhaps herpes would be an interesting experience." But there is so little we understand about biologic terrain that our terrain could easily be expressing activating information to latent viruses in our system.

Why would some aspect of us choose an illness? This "choice" only makes sense when we return to a more spiritual understanding of physical existence. There is always a reason that illness occurs. We are not being punished by illness. We are here as expressions of love. Our bodies are made of love. The choice of our body to accept illness always indicates that our physical selves are somehow limiting or obstructing the flow of love that is really who we are. The actual illness is a mirror of our lack of flow. It is a vehicle allowing me to show myself some aspect, pattern, or behavior that I have overlooked.

The bodymindspirit chooses illness as the best route, in the current moment, to get us back into the flow of love, the best way to remind us of our greater selves, the best way to illustrate our misconceptions so we can release them.

For example, genital herpes, HSV type 2, is a virus that colonizes humans. In most infected people it is dormant most of the time. In my experience, its activity level is a reliable indicator of stress. There is never "no reason" why a herpes infection flares. Perhaps general feelings of discomfort with sexuality or more specific feelings about our sexual expression with a particular partner modify the terrain to be more favorable to uncoating the genital herpes virus in some people. Perhaps there has been overindulgence in food or drink. Perhaps there has been fighting, or financial stressors. When people have frequent outbreaks, I encourage them to examine feelings about sexuality, relationship, body image, and physical contact, and to look at general life stressors as well.

Perhaps, on a similar note, an ongoing low-level stress, or the stress of insufficient sleep, or mixed feelings about what one is eating or drinking or doing with one's life contribute to a terrain favorable to a common cold. The net result of a viral infection may be that we slow down and rest. This is a good thing. It gives us time to think a bit, and to consider what might be up for us.

Viruses that are pathogenic, meaning they cause illness, are generally only problematic for one species, or a group of related species. Tobacco mosaic virus, for example, affects plants in the nicotiana family but is harmless for humans, animals, and all other types of plants.

Even bacteria have their own viruses, called bacteriophages. This knowledge has already resulted in a cooperative venture between people and certain viruses. A type of treatment developed in Russia, called phage therapy, employs these bacterial-specific viruses as an alternative to antibiotics. Because the phages only affect specific bacteria, they can be selected and utilized for specific organisms.

Bacteriophages do not infect human or animal cells, so a bacterio-phage chosen for its ability to penetrate salmonella would have no adverse consequences for the helpful acidophilus and bifidus colonies of our intestinal tracts but could easily help us to swiftly clear a sal-monella infection. Further study of phage therapy is one promising arena for exploration and cooperation with the viral world. Perhaps an even better model would include and value the consciousness of the salmonella bacteria in the conversation.

Like bacterial infections, viruses will affect individuals in different ways. For example, hepatitis B is a virus that causes damage to the liver. In most people, the virus causes an acute illness, which can be mild or severe, then the immune system overcomes it and the person recovers fully. Afterwards, the affected individual is permanently im-mune to hepatitis B. But approximately five percent of adults who contract hepatitis B will go on to become chronic carriers of the dis-ease. They can infect others with it, and their own health may con-tinue to be affected. Long-term infection with hepatitis B may be asymptomatic or may lead to chronic hepatitis, cirrhosis of the liver, and even liver cancer. Hepatitis B is prevalent in large portions of the world. It is estimated that three to six percent of the Earth's human population harbors the hepatitis B virus and more than one-third of the population has been exposed to it at some time in their life.

Viruses that we consider pathological tend to replicate when we are weaker. In this they can be said to be opportunists and/or can be seen as providing information about our overall state of being. I could have included viruses in the upcoming chapter on messengers, since their activation conveys important information about our over-all state of self-alignment and well-being. Any microorganism that interacts with humans can play a messengerial role. The question is, can we hear and interpret the message? When we feel we are vic-timized by illness, then we miss the self-awareness opportunity and resultant growth that can ensue from the energetic exchange. If we understand, however, that an infection is not a personal affront but a road map pointing to greater flourishing, then we have tuned in to the alchemy inherent in any illness, and we are on the road to positive transformation.

In researching viruses, I was amazed to see that it appears that no one has considered viruses in other than three ways:

1. How can they harm us, or our extensions (our crops, animals, etc.)?
2. How can we destroy or inactivate them?
3. How can we exploit them with technologies like genetic modification?

What are possible benefits of viruses? Well, we know viruses are one way in which nature can introduce new genetic material into an existing organism. This process is called transduction, considered to be one of the factors, along with spontaneous mutation, that supports evolutionary change.

Now imagine that instead of all this being random, it is anything but that. Viruses could be instruments of rapid and meaningful exchange of genetic information among organisms. We know, for example, that plasmids—virus-like molecules of DNA that exist and replicate separately from host DNA—are a main route for transfer of information between bacteria about antibiotic resistance. Viruses and their sister proto-life forms, plasmids, can be very positive evolutionarily, introducing whole chunks of genetic material in a very short time, even within a lifetime. This is far-fetched to people who believe evolution occurs in a slow, laborious manner, as most of us were taught in elementary school. Still, our understanding about plasmids and viruses exonerates the much maligned and ridiculed contemporary of Darwin, Jean-Baptiste Lamarck. Lamarck believed individuals could pass on to their offspring characteristics that they acquired during their lives. On a cellular level, through mechanisms such as plasmid-mediated DNA transmission, Lamarck's theories are now understood to be absolutely true.

The narrow understanding of the theory of evolution, despite remaining widely promoted, has been essentially disproved. There are no anthropologic or fossil records of intermediate species that classical Darwinism predicts. According to the actual fossil record, eons pass on Earth with species exhibiting stability and little change. Evolution appears to happen in rapid bursts, in exceedingly short periods of time. The Cambrian explosion that led to the immense diversity of life on our planet would not have been possible by the slow model of evolutionary growth. Researchers believe that viruses have played a key role during periods of rapid evolutionary growth in development of new species. That we do not know how or why this occurs indicates that perhaps we have not been asking the right questions, or basing our inquiry on the right premises.

Let's start again with some of our new premises, specifically that:

a. Love is the fundamental basis of reality, the fabric of which everything is woven.
b. All matter has consciousness. Consciousness is always expanding, moving toward greater love.
c. There is a bigger picture of non-physical reality. We are a portion of non-physical reality and entirely contained within it.

Then: In the service of that love, viruses most likely have important, even essential roles to play. This is most readily seen in their capacity for transformation of life. While this is speculative, I believe it is the case, and there is evidence in modern science to support this notion.

Viruses, for example, are currently used extensively in genetic engineering, as they easily penetrate cell walls. Engineered viruses can transport segments of genetic information into a cell envelope, and they can be coded so the genetic information they contain will be incorporated at specific points in the host genome.

Because of our society's current distrustful attitude toward viruses, I am especially wary of genetically modified organisms and crops (GMOs). Utilizing viruses to transfer parts of the genome of one type of organism to another is one way to create GMOs. Like it or not, we are rapidly developing in laboratories a host of new genetically engineered species, such as tomatoes with salmon DNA and cattle with human genes inserted to produce milk that is similar to human milk.[2] But we have not exactly arrived at a peaceful place with these proto-organisms. Most people have more positive feelings for crystals and minerals than they do for viruses.

On the positive side, this means there are tremendous opportunities ahead of us for collaboration and cooperation, based upon mutual respect. But I imagine that the resultant efforts will be very different from the products of the current science of exploitation. I find genetic engineering as a product of reductionist industrial-driven science fairly disconcerting, precisely because there is no one listening to the voice of nature.

Nature, however, is certainly speaking. For example, in pregnant herd animals fed certain GMO crops, up to forty-five percent experience miscarriage, and twenty percent are infertile. This may be due to the presence of a novel pathogen in the crops, or to the high levels of pesticide to which the animals are exposed via the ingested plant material, or some other mechanism.[3,4] The pathogen and the fertility problem have not been observed in animals eating wild grasses or organic feed.

With a new awareness, healthy respect, and new practices that evolve from these, it is certain that we will befriend and cooperatively create with viruses, plasmids, and a host of other organisms and proto-organisms in balanced and mutually agreeable ways. For example, as humans move out into the stars and live on new planets, we will undoubtedly engage in some amount of terraforming of amenable habitable worlds. This has been predicted in science fiction since the beginning of the genre. Many other ideas that are now "reality," including Earth-orbiting satellites, credit cards, robots, touch-screen technology, and cloning, emerged first in the medium of science fiction, so it is entirely reasonable to believe that terraforming other planets might eventually be a reality. Viruses, I believe, will be essential intermediaries in the transfer of information about the future inhabitants to the cooperative planetary body that is welcoming life.

I imagine there is much research to do examining the life-enhancing and beneficial properties of viruses. But they might need to be renamed. If viruses are really a cosmic type of messenger/delivery service, then we might prefer to name them after Hermes, messenger of the gods. We could call them hermions, a pleasant word connoting their messengerial functions, which also has some vague hermaphroditic sexual overtones that the particles themselves would surely appreciate. Like Hermes, they are fast and expedient. They enormously simplify complex tasks including the fundamental shifting of life forms. In my interactions with them in the Silver World, viruses have a fun, "can-do" attitude.

In physics we thought we had it all down when we discovered atoms, then found particles, then learned that electrons, neutrons, and protons are made of even tinier particles like hadrons and quarks. Recently experiments from the Large Hadron Collider at CERN have intimated that the most fundamental particle, the Higgs boson, may really be five particles.[5] It appears in physics that any new answer brings many new questions. The biological sciences are no different. Nature's tapestry is infinite.

I previously described some of my experience of the Golden World. When there, I understand that we are all one. I see here and now is eternally a unified whole. In that state of consciousness, I understand that there is no Other that we must learn to trust because there are no others. Only an eternal "I" exists. We all have access to the Golden World; each of us can know our oneness with all reality.

I acknowledge that while those are lovely insights for moments of mystical contemplation, we are here, in this "real" world. In our physical world, of course, there appear to be others—billions of other humans, millions of dolphins, hundreds of billions of birds among more than ten thousand species, innumerable insects, and unfathomable numbers of bacteria, spores, and viruses. Amazing others surround us, like silkworms, tarantulas, house moths, wasps, and gazelles. There are simple one-celled Others, and complex thinking organisms with the ability to use tools and to solve problems, such as raccoons, parrots, and chimpanzees. The word "animal" itself comes from the Latin *anima*, meaning spirit, or breath of life. That there is only one anima, only one breath of life, is something we may not often consider as we swim in this sea of diversity.

We can direct our focus and we can control our thoughts. We can shift our image of what we see by looking in a different direction, or seeing the same things in a new light. The meaning of events in our lives is determined by our beliefs. As we grow to trust that life is meaningful, we appreciate our experiences for what they offer us and teach us about ourselves. Sometimes it is good to merely breathe and recall for a moment that the breath of life is the same in all of us, including viruses. While our lives are very different and multitudinous, life force is one. This simple action helps us root into our heart and perceive in a different way than the busy brain alone allows us. It reminds us that all physical matter is spiritual matter, and that we already know, inside ourselves, our essential oneness. Trust arises from our hearts.

We can notice, through observation of the effects of the Law of Attraction, that everything we experience matches our own vibration. Trust eventually becomes an understanding of self. We trust ourselves to be reliable and to allow our highest good. We trust ourselves to find the best way. We trust our cells and organs to admit and uncoat viruses for a greater good, in the service of the love that we are.

Sometimes this means flourishing health, when we are flowing life force through ourselves without obstruction. Sometimes this means illness to call us back into balance. We can bless and respect viruses and plasmids. They too are sacred. They too are my self. There are no Others.

Tools for Transformation

Consider these questions:

1. How do I feel about viruses?
2. Do viruses show me anything about myself right now?
3. How do they teach us alignment with the great field of Love?
4. Are viruses emblematic of my feelings of trust or lack of it?
5. How does the idea of cooperation with them feel to me?

Now imagine some scenarios where viruses and humans playfully co-create. Tell a story to yourself of viruses and kindness.

The next time you have a cold or flu, or are beginning to exhibit symptoms, try a dialogue with the virus similar to the one mentioned in the previous exercise on Lyme or bacteria.

1. Does this virus have something to tell me about myself?
2. Could it be a divine messenger? What could the message be?
3. Speak to the virus as you would a friend, and listen as if hearing the thoughts of a beloved and trusted advisor.
4. Record any insights in your journal. Be aware that more may come at a later time.

—CHAPTER TEN—
Messengers

N EW QUESTIONS SPROUT UP LIKE daffodils in spring as we begin to comprehend that the natural world is constantly communicating with us. The big picture of a changed awareness of reality might seem overwhelming at first. To make the matter simpler, one might wisely begin to approach nature on a personal level. A good jumping-off point is asking, "What do interconnectedness and vibration mean for me personally and for my understanding of my own health concerns?" I encourage this line of inquiry in my patients. Real health comes from creating balance within ourselves. We must address our own inner harmony in order to thrive as individuals and to create greater well-being in our society and civilization.

We get novel personal answers to old questions—like why some people sicken when exposed to a bacteria, fungus, or virus while others remain healthy—by seeing ourselves anew as beings living every facet of our lives within a web of significant relationships. Understanding dawns about why illness comes gently to some and in a raging fury to others. Illness is meaningful on an individual level and on a systemic level.

When I was a third-year medical student, the first patient death I experienced was that of a ninety-four-year-old gentleman I'll call Joseph. He had lived a remarkably healthy and happy life. On his intake history and physical Joseph was amiable, joking playfully with the staff and me. Joseph told us his philosophy of life had always been to live life to the fullest by spending his time doing things he loved. He was too "lazy" to spend time in boring or unpleasant activities, so he had passionately pursued joy in all areas of his life. He was easy-going and loved lots of things like family, travel, golf, and theatre. Joseph had opened his own travel business when he was young so he would be able to see more of the world. This had turned into a financially successful venture. He had officially retired many years earlier and still continued doing the things he loved, including advising two of his grandchildren who now ran the travel agency.

Joseph had been well until the morning prior to his hospital admission, though he had been feeling "very sleepy" for about a week. He had no major illnesses but was "getting tired" and felt he was "winding down." He was at peace with this notion, especially since his wife of more than seventy years had passed away around six months earlier. He awakened the previous day feeling a little under the weather and had noticed a cough. This grew worse through the day. His family was concerned so they brought him to the hospital early the next morning. He had many children, grandchildren, and great-grandchildren and was loved and respected by all of them. Joseph was swiftly diagnosed with pneumonia, and we started him on antibiotics, cough medication, and oxygen. These helped his comfort level greatly, alleviating the symptoms he had developed. He spent the remainder of the day alternating between rests and jovially visiting with family members.

Joseph died in his sleep in the wee hours of the next morning without any significant suffering. He had been driving his car the week before his illness. His family really appreciated how easy his dying had been. It seemed to befit the kind, happy, and caring person he had been in this life. The pneumococcal bacteria came gently, and when he was ready, they eased him from life. It was easy to see why, in medicine, pneumococcus is sometimes called "the old man's friend." It was clear that this bacteria was a friend, not an enemy. His family members were grateful that he had passed so quickly and painlessly, experiencing only minor discomfort for less than forty-eight hours. His granddaughter and I talked and agreed it was among the gentlest of deaths. She could not have wished anything easier and milder for her beloved grandpa. The whole family was remarkable and filled with his same spirit. Even in his death they celebrated his life. I was amazed that no one seemed upset.

In retrospect, it is not surprising to me that Joseph was the first patient who died while I was caring for him. I have always been comfortable with physical death because of my clear experiential knowledge that we are eternal beings. I have always understood that physical death is a passage, a doorway between understandings. I have been able to communicate with those who have crossed its threshold since I was small, though I shared this gift with only a few people until recently. The way the simplicity and comfort of his death experience matched the beauty and ease of his life gave me an important lesson. Tales of great spiritual masters who transit consciously from their physical body have always fascinated me. Joseph's peaceful death, after a full and happy life, was as close to one of those transcendent deaths as any I had previously experienced first-hand.

Although occurring in a hospital, this death seemed utterly natural to me. Like animals or insects dying, there was no fear in Joseph, and no particular struggle or suffering. It was a hint of something available to any of us, and I stored this gem of understanding away to unpack at a later date.

On the other hand, most contemporary humans struggle with illness and even more so with death. Illnesses are feared as out-of-control and random forces, rather than being acknowledged as gentle, meaningful friends. When illness seems other than a kind and benevolent ally, we can reframe this limited understanding by examining the models nature provides. Nature helps us understand the complex web of intercommunication and interdependency that characterizes our lives. Nature helps us see health and illness as eloquent vehicles of communication and cooperation that lead to greater thriving for the whole of who we are.

In a forest fungi, bacteria, and viruses will occupy and eventually consume the life of an ill tree. The tree might be ill for a number of reasons. It may have become damaged by a storm or may be too shaded by other trees. It may have been weakened by the actions of humans, animals, or birds; or it might be growing in soil too deficient in nutrients. Whatever the reason, the sick tree emits chemical messages including pheromones that invite bacteria, fungi, and insects to nourish themselves on its tissue. It is as if the tree says to the other organisms responsible for degradation and decay, "Come and get me, because it is time to recycle this physical matter into the big pool of matter." Even parts of trees do this. If a whole tree is healthy but a limb is weak, then just that branch will emit the pheromones and the rest of the tree will withdraw its nourishing energy from the damaged part. It will isolate the area from the rest of the healthy tissue, sealing it off even as it invites organisms of decomposition to dine on the frail branch.

Among animals, as with plants, insects, and trees, it is usually the weak, the vulnerable, and the frail that become dinner for other animals. Perhaps there is a communication between predator and accessible prey in the dance of life. Predatory animals easily recognize the injured prey, the old one, and the one who is ill and unable to keep up with the others. These are easier to catch and there is a natural recycling.

There are more examples of organisms in nature communicating about health and illness. Essential to understanding this communication is the knowledge that no other organisms are afraid of death. They wither and try to avoid suffering, as do humans, but animals do not fight death when it is time. Animals will run away from danger, fleeing and fighting when they believe there is a chance for escape, but they surrender when they know the game is over. They relax and let go. Organisms will try to thrive as best they can and enjoy their day in the sun. They are great teachers of living life to the fullest, and they let go easily when it is clear that days of life in a particular body have passed. A happy and loved domestic cat will often hide from its human companions when it knows death is near. Some intentionally put themselves in harm's way. I know of many cats that have gone out and seemingly deliberately been struck by cars when they were old and sick. The cat, unlike its human companions, does not perceive death as something to be avoided at all costs.

Ants will risk their lives exploring new food and water sources for their colony. It is part of their nature as cooperative communal insects. An injured ant sends out particular signals, and nurse ants will attend to it for healing if they are able. However, nurse ants will not waste energy attending to an ant that is too far gone. Everything ants do is for the good of the community.

It is likely that one reason we become fatally colonized by bacteria or infected by fungus or virus is due to mechanisms similar to the damaged tree branch. When we are weak or frail or very elderly, there is a natural recycling. We do not like to think of death this way, and for most of us such an "allowing" of disease is certainly without our conscious awareness. I was recently reading about the upsurge of hospital-acquired infections. The article explained that the very elderly, those over eighty-five years old, were at greatest risk of dying of these infections. "Well, duh!" I thought. "Is this necessarily a bad thing?" The very elderly generally die at a higher rate than the young. Actuarial tables certainly affirm this observation. Many of us view it as a tragedy when a young person dies. But as a society, we have a real problem if we think it is a tragedy when any person dies at any age, because, of course, every person will die. The chance of mortality is one hundred percent.

I believe the ideal—but rarely achieved—way to die is the method of spiritual masters. It is simply to be done with all one has to do for this life and to leave one's body. After living a full life like Joseph's it is possible, at any age, to feel ready to transition to something else, knowing death is just a doorway, a shift in perspective. I have subsequently known other patients and friends who died peacefully, aware of their true nature. They were ready for a fresh perspective. It is truly uplifting to be with these people physically and spiritually as they make their transition.

In most of us death is an unconscious process. Our cells are aware, though, of the need for transformation, even if our limited mind is not. How does the cell know it is time to sicken or die, either as an individual part or as a whole organism? There are messages sent and messages received. We can be more consciously aware of both sides of this communication when we understand that communication to and from the rest of the natural world is occurring.

For example, when there is an infection, there are many subtle and overt messages that microorganisms receive. Bacteria often navigate their environment by chemotaxis, a chemically mediated impulse of motion toward or away from certain biochemical signals. Our immune cells also migrate by chemotaxis to the site of an infection, to clear up debris that might be emitting a "come and get me" message, and to engulf and deactivate bacteria who have come in response to that message. When our immune system is healthy, it can easily handle the load, effectively saying to the bacteria, "never mind" or "not now." Cells, like trees, animals, and insects, also broadcast chemical messages as pheromones advertising the existing situation to interested parties.

Now think of the smells in a hospital or a sickroom. There is often, of course, disinfectant, which masks some of the other olfactory sensations. Besides this, there is usually an odor of human decay. As we grow more infirm, we, like the trees, also emit chemical messages that say, "Come and get me." These messages signal to bacteria, fungi, and other organisms that a ready food source is nearby. Organisms of human decay naturally accumulate in regions like hospitals, where there is more food for them. Whether we like it or not, hospitals are repositories of some of the most powerful and hardy strains of bacteria. The more we develop tools to try to fight them, the stronger they get. They are not going away because they are an essential part of the overall balance of life.

Once there are greater concentrations of bacteria and immune cells that are trying to break them down, we get more pungent and overt smells—those of pus, rot, and putrefaction. These odors are neither good nor bad. While they smell unpleasant, they are just information and communication. In someone who is very ill, the forces of decomposition will outbalance the forces of repair. The individual may die of "overwhelming sepsis" which means generalized infection all over the body. There is no ambiguity to the message the bacteria are receiving in this instance. Instead, it's time for them to feast and to multiply.

It is interesting to note that while we may be afraid of death, the cells of our body are not. The cells themselves are emitting the chemical messages inviting the bacteria. Our cells, as we saw in the previous chapter, may even choose to activate latent viruses. When we are very ill, our cells are ready to let go of this life and move on, allowing the nutrients of our physical vehicle to be recycled into another life form.

Chemical and electrical messages from our own cells to other areas of our body also activate processes like inflammation and accelerated cell growth of cancers. Contemporary medical science thinks of these as pathological, but they are simply other mediators that expedite the process of transformation that sometimes includes death. When our immune system is overwhelmed for any reason, we succumb to illness.

Communication is a back and forth, a call and response. If we do not like what we are receiving in response, then it is helpful to examine what we might be communicating. Remember that most communication, including human-to-human communication, is nonverbal. As our language incorrectly assumes that we are at war with the natural world, we might erroneously perceive that we are under attack if we have an infection or another ailment, even an undesired growth like a cancer. If the natural world is, in fact, communicating with us, mirroring our vibrational output, then it would be helpful for us to look gently and lovingly at ourselves and to ask what messages we are transmitting in the form of expectations, beliefs, emotions, and focus of thoughts.

Our bodies are part of the natural world. We have a physical body, but we are not merely this body. Most of us are not aware that we are communicating at every moment. The majority of humans do not know what messages they are transmitting, as most of us have never asked that question of ourselves. Many of us are not in touch with our feelings at all and have no comprehension that our emotional state, our focus, and our thoughts are forms of communication. How our emotions feel to us, the level of ease or discomfort, gives us important messages about the broadcast we are offering. When we are aware of how we feel, we notice that it always feels best to have peaceful, joyous, harmonious, and calm emotions. But sometimes we are unaware of how we feel. This is often the case when there is an ongoing pattern. We begin to ignore and then completely stop noticing feelings of discomfort from unresolved thoughts and actions.

Recently, I realized that a cluster of symptoms I had had for a long time was actually a chronic sinus infection—probably part bacterial and part fungal. In the past I would have regarded this as something that just "happened." But I know too much. Illness does not just happen. Something that I was offering up unintentionally was contributing to the health problem that was now occurring. I did not feel blameful or victimized. The awareness came when I was able to be interested in how I might shift myself toward greater thriving. If anything, I found myself amused by the situation.

The deeper meaning of the symptoms I exhibited with the sinus infection might have been easily interpreted, if I had been paying attention while it was evolving. My first sign was a headache above my right eye. Was there pain in how I was seeing things? Yes, but I did not ask the question at that stage. The next sign was a weeping discharge from my right eye. Were some of my beliefs, some of my ways of looking at the world making me sad, causing tears? Yes, but I still did not understand. I kept thinking, "What is wrong with me?" At times I would silently catastrophize, thinking thoughts such as "Could I have a brain tumor?" although ninety-nine percent of me knew this was absurd. My head would hurt more when I ate sweets or drank wine, things I did not feel whole-hearted about. I would eat or drink these even as I said to myself, "I know this isn't good for me." My body kindly obliged with head pain as an instant manifestation of my disconnection with myself. I often explain to patients that we are eating not only foods but also the thoughts we think about them. If I have a donut and think, "I should not eat this, it is bad for me" then I am setting up an expectation of something undesired that is sure to materialize. I am priming the pump of my subconscious to seek evidence of something I do not want yet expect to occur.

Whenever I thought about the sinus and head symptoms, I felt annoyance or fear, both very familiar emotions. There was a perfect vibrational match between the manifestation of illness and my self-defeating thought patterns. So why was I still not getting it? Essentially because these habits of thought were so embedded that I no longer noticed them. Eventually I looked at how the illness made me feel, since emotional response to illness is often a clue about what got it started in the first place. This is a useful tool of self-examination I learned from Abraham-Hicks that I have employed countless times with my patients and myself. Since the symptoms had been mildly occurring for quite a while, I knew the thoughts and focus contributing to it were probably familiar things. Here was my cooperative body, amplifying the dysfunctional pattern so I would ideally begin to attend to it. Emotionally, my response to the infection was a feeling of not being good enough, feeling disappointed and frustrated that circumstances of my life were seemingly not in my control. I also felt ashamed that I, a teacher of healthy living, had an ongoing health problem.

One day the pain intensified to a level where I was unable to focus upon anything else, and drainage of yellow pus (apologies for the gross-out) began to weep from the corner of my right eye. While I knew it was time for antibiotics, I finally connected the dots of what my body was saying to me. The situation was festering. I used antibiotics as a tool in the restoration of my balance. But the balance itself came from my finally hearing what I was communicating and what the bacteria and fungi were mirroring back to me.

My emotional responses gave me a lot to go on, and I looked for where else in my life I might be feeling similar things and projecting similar thoughts. The answers became apparent almost as soon as I inquired. Looking at myself I noticed that I had habits of thought that did not serve my greater good. I had self-deprecating thoughts. I felt sad and inadequate over simple things. I frequently compared myself to others and judged myself harshly. For example, I went to a friend's house and admired their garden. I could have said internally, "Wow, what a lovely garden! It has a great design, nice flow, and a rich color palette. How inspiring!" Instead I chose to feel bad about myself. I compared my garden achievements to my friend's and then I judged myself unworthy, rather than feeling the delight, inspiration, and appreciation their garden offered.

I had also continued to ride a roller coaster of feeling "too fat" and often gazed at my body with dissatisfaction rather than love. Even though I work with patients to help them shift these exact same beliefs, I had to acknowledge that I was not free of them myself. I saw that my negative habits of thought were more pervasive than I wanted to admit. They were festering. Once I identified them, I knew I could begin to shift. It didn't matter how they began or why I had ongoing self-critical internal banter. All I needed was the awareness of what I was offering to the cosmic instant-messaging service and the desire to feel better. In this case feeling better meant greater self-acceptance, greater inner harmony, and more enjoyment. It meant genuinely feeling good about my body, whatever its size. I could whole-heartedly embrace these goals and ask my inner guidance for assistance in noticing and shifting my self-defeating thoughts and beliefs.

I elected not to take an antifungal medication because the severe pain was relieved after the antibiotic. I knew the opportunity to love myself more would be enhanced by working consciously in conjunction with the remaining microbes to restore balance. I wanted to eat in harmony with what my body was asking, and to think positive thoughts when I had a meal or snack. I saw that I had long desired to notice and shift the negative self-talk and finally acknowledged this to myself. I also felt ready to drop judgments about other people, especially unsolicited judgments about what they eat. While I still give advice when people request it, now advice begins with helping people connect with their own sense of well-being and honest alignment with themselves. While a patient or I might eventually want to change a particular dietary habit, it is much easier to do so from a place of self-acceptance. One major step is to eat only foods that feel good in the moment we intend to consume them. This means being aware of what we are thinking about the food as we eat it. When we can internally say and believe constructive statements about our foods, then we are in alignment with our highest good. It is not that a brownie or ice cream is bad or good in and of itself. Rather, eating the thought "this is bad for me, I should not have it" over and over again, as many of us do, drives us toward outcomes we both deplore and expect.

Obviously, shifting how we do something as fundamental as eating is a process that takes time, patience, and humor. It involves slowing down and paying attention. It involves believing in yourself and allowing your higher good. With a new awareness, I can skip the brownie for now, or change my thoughts to self-loving ones and go ahead and eat it if it feels okay. As I applied this new way of thinking and acting, over time I relaxed. My sinuses improved greatly. I now spend more time seeking and observing evidence of health in my patients, my family, my world, and myself. I continue retraining myself to attend to minor feelings of disconnection and discomfort in response to inharmonious thoughts, rather than waiting for dramatic indicators to present themselves. I let myself be playful and indulgent through all of this. We build healthful practices when we shift to greater self-awareness through kindness. Berating ourselves for falling into old traps is never useful.

Three things I find most helpful in creating new life-affirming patterns are to a) look without judgment at what I am communicating, b) notice how I am communicating it and how my cooperative body is mirroring me to myself, and c) affirm a new thought that reflects the self-love I know in my heart. I can then look at the bacteria and fungus in my sinuses in a different way and appreciate how they were amplifying my own discomfort and dis-ease for me. I had put out a small "come and get me" message and they had graciously obliged. This became an excellent co-creation in service of my greater harmony. I did not blame them for "invading" me. I understood they were there at my invitation, shining a spotlight on habits of thought so ingrained that I had stopped paying attention to them long ago.

When we are a little bit ill, like I was with my persistent sinus infection, it is often because we are transmitting mixed signals. Though usually I felt good about myself, I was thinking too often: "I am not good, I am not worthy, life is dissatisfying." The universe responded lovingly to my messages by demonstrating my pain and contradictions to me. While messages come to us in many ways, the body is an excellent vehicle for nature, spirit, and our inner guidance to communicate with us because we care so much about it. Our body and our health easily attract our attention when they are off balance.

Minor or fleeting thoughts that are not aligned with our true nature of love might give us a moment of discomfort, a gripping in the stomach, or a tightening in the shoulders. We can train ourselves to be more sensitive to these subtle cues from our body about what we are transmitting to the greater whole. One question I ask almost every patient is "Where in your body do you put your stress?" In more than twenty years of medical practice, I have met only a handful of patients who could not immediately identify where he or she parked upsetting thoughts and emotions. Most people have been trained to ignore or misinterpret the little messages they get, even from their self-acknowledged areas of tension, so eventually the messages get louder and more insistent.

When there is a minor viral illness, it's often because we have temporarily overworked or pushed ourselves too hard. We have not been paying attention to balance in our life or listening to our inner wisdom. In doing so, we unconsciously emit messages that invite viruses already present in us to replicate and invite new viruses to join them. We indicate to our cells that it is time for dormant viruses to uncoat and express themselves. For example, how many college students do you know who drive themselves furiously to get through finals, then come home for a break and spend the next two weeks down with the flu?

When we have an acute infection, the body is asking to come back into balance. Balance is not a quick fix to mask symptoms in order to push on. Our college student lacks sleep and is trying to live on a diet of sweets and caffeine. He "knows" this isn't good for him but does it anyway because he feels he has no choice. He spends much of his time inefficiently trying to cram in information. He may be feeling overwhelmed and thinking mildly discouraging thoughts such as "I don't know if I can pull this off." All the while a tiny voice inside is asking for rest, a more relaxed, serene type of study, and real nutrition. But that voice is ignored. "I don't have time," he tells himself, "to meditate, sleep, or cook a good meal." The student's body knows otherwise. His mind does not efficiently process information with all the pressure and lack of ease. Adrenaline drives him through finals week, but after exams, when the fear-, caffeine-, and sugar-fueled rush is over, he finds himself exhausted. Ideally the resulting infection, fatigue, or illness helps the student to slow down, to listen inwardly, and to rest.

Generally we misinterpret what is occurring because our beliefs—supported by our culture and social cues—say that this is all "random." We still may not be ready or able to pay attention. The student thinks to himself, "I must have picked up a bug," instead of considering that "a virus was my body's amplification of its loud but ignored request for more rest and more self-caring."

I often talk to students about studying smarter. We learn better when we are refreshed, relaxed, and well-nourished. We retain little that we cram in. Just the word "cram" implies scarcity of space and tightness. Students who try a relaxed approach, even at finals time, see immediately that it is more effective. We retain and easily access much more data learned in a low-stress or stress-free environment. The hours of study undertaken when well rested are worth many times as much as bleary-eyed strain. Plus, when we are well rested we are more in touch with our intuitive capacity. We can more naturally flow our attention to things that feel important and that might actually be important for our exams or for our creative output.

Sustained inharmonious emotions weaken our immune system and allow various organisms and pathologic conditions to gain a foothold. For example, there was a study done in which African American volunteers had a number of immune parameters in their blood checked when they were at rest and feeling calm. Immediately afterwards they were subjected to a barrage of racist remarks. (I wonder as I write this: who funds these studies and why would anyone volunteer for them?) When the subjects' blood was tested just after the remarks, the immune activity had decreased significantly.[1] This was a short-term test in volunteers who knew what was being studied. How much greater are the effects on the immune system when we are sad, fearful, up-set, or angry much of the time as a result of real-life stressors? What if we go through life with our predominant everyday emotions not supporting well-being? What happens to the immune system then?

The immune system is physiologically keyed to well-being. When we are happy it hums along efficiently. When we are acutely stressed, immune activity takes a nose-dive. When we have chronic tension, many things go awry immunologically since our predominant emo-tions may include feelings of loneliness, anger, victimization, resent-ment, or fear. Then we are the injured prey, transmitting that our cells are available to other elements of the natural world for transforma-tion and recycling.

The industrial medical response to illness is to treat the symptoms of illness while ignoring the message. If we have a cold, we take medi-cines that dry us up. If we have heartburn, we are prescribed medi-cines that block acid production. If we have allergies we are given anti-histamines, powerful systemic medications that block release of a key compound in the inflammatory/secretory chain of events. We call all effects of such medications that are not directly shifting our symptom "side effects," but they are not peripheral; they are addi-tional effects. Anti-histamines, for example, are systemic drugs that will make us drowsy, cause dry mucous membranes, and slow our digestion, causing bloating.

Homeopathic perspective says that illness is driven deeper into the body by treatments that only address symptoms instead of the underlying causes. Treating a skin problem with steroids or cutting out a small tumor does not end the imbalance. The problem will pop up in a more aggressive form at a later date if the underlying imbal-ance is not corrected. Surgery or pharmaceuticals can be helpful tools, but they are best utilized in a larger context. If the underlying cause is a vibrational pattern, a misunderstanding, then the vibrational pattern that caused the problem is ultimately what needs to be corrected.

Years ago I had a patient with a severe case of psoriasis. It covered parts of her face and much of her arms. We tried many tools to correct it and these would work for a while, but eventually the problem would return full-force. This puzzled me, so we gently explored her feelings about the psoriasis. She thought her skin condition made her look "ugly" and "freakish" but also admitted that it gave her a barrier to others and made her feel safe. When the psoriasis was active she was less likely to be touched, and she realized she felt quite vulnerable when it was not present. It turned out that she had experienced incest as a child. She had known this and thought she "had worked through it," so had never connected the incest and her feelings of vulnerability with her psoriasis. She and I agreed it was pointless at that time to try to "cure" a skin condition that was the only thing helping her maintain a sense of safe boundaries. She entered into somatic psychotherapy to develop a greater sense of ease in the world, and liked it so much that she decided to become a somatic psychotherapist.

I saw her again, several years later. She was a different and much happier individual. She had good self-esteem, healthy boundaries, and was in a loving relationship with a compassionate man who really understood her. She had confidence about her safety in the world. Her skin was better without any remedies, natural or pharmaceutical. We were easily able to clear up most of the remnants of the problem with some dietary changes and herbal support. She still has bouts of mild psoriasis but has learned to work with this manifestation and notice minor feelings of vulnerability and fearfulness before the problem gets very big. She actually enjoys the opportunity for honest, non-judgmental self-examination that her skin condition affords her, greeting it with a willingness to embody a greater wholeness, greater self-love, and greater inner and outer peace.

Often I observe patients whose illness becomes a focal point of fear and worry, a disconnection that leads to expansion of "pathological" conditions in an effort of the soul to bring the message of a return to balance to a crescendo. When we are seriously ill or feel miserable, we are living in extreme dis-ease, and we send loud messages to the natural world that we are ready for colonization and other ailments. Nature always obliges. We have all been around people who are very ill. Not only is there the odor of decay, there also is a bioenergetic vibration that cheerful colors cannot mask.

I propose we look at all of this differently. What if we considered the presence of imbalanced bacteria or an illness as a response message rather than an affront? What if we understood that we are co-creators and not victims? What if the manifestation of illness were really just a part of the process of healing, of restoring balance, orchestrated from the level of our soul? What if we thought of illness as a way that consciousness is communicating with us—indeed, responding to our own bioenergetic messages? This different understanding of illness is the foundation from which a new understanding of health and illness can be built. If we assume that the universe is love, and that everything that comes to us emanates from that love, then illness, however unpleasant or seemingly awful, flows from and serves that same love, offering us an opportunity to make choices that enable us to live as fuller expressions of our souls.

In nature, when all the individuals in a herd are healthy, the predators still need to eat. Then the one who separates itself from the pack is eaten. The balance of life depends upon the well-being of the whole community. Could it be deliberate that a vigorous young gazelle that becomes food for the lion is responding to some inner urge to support the balance of life? While this seems far-fetched to our modern sensibilities, it is in fact what people of traditional cultures worldwide report.

In Native American tribes of the Great Plains, a prayer was always said before the buffalo hunt. The buffalo that separated itself from the herd was the one harvested by the tribe. That separation was an indication of a gift the animal was making of its life. It was understood to be the response of the Great Buffalo Spirit to the request of the hunters for nourishment and sustenance for the people. The buffalo hunt was an integral and sacred part of Plains Indian culture, and after the buffalo was taken, virtually all parts of it were used for food, medicine, clothing, or shelter. The few unusable bits were returned to the earth.

Like the buffalo that separates itself from the herd to nourish humans in the great cycle of life, perhaps there are some people who, from the level of their soul and knowing their eternal nature, become ill and even die to point the way toward awareness of a need for correction of great societal imbalance. These individuals self-select from a higher level of consciousness, lovingly indicating our societal vibrational discrepancies through the gift of their life experiences.

What about the innocent? Why do bad things seemingly happen to good people? It might be possible to reframe, in this context, the illnesses of "innocent" beings, like babies born with congenital defects, or small children with cancers like leukemia. For example, could rising rates of childhood cancers be related to our disquiet with the increasingly prevalent disruptive electromagnetic fields circulating our planet, fields that affect us and all other life? Could they relate to our dis-ease with our culture generating mounting levels of persistent nuclear waste, or to other environmental damage from industrialization? Or might they relate to some other aspect of our dominant culture with which we have collectively overlooked our disharmony?

Perhaps, too, infants with serious congenital conditions might really be the embodiment of great spiritual teachers offering humanity opportunities for unconditional love. Consider, for example, how very loving, sweet, and "pure" many people with Down's syndrome seem to be. The deeply moving book *Expecting Adam* was written by the parent of one such Down's syndrome child. Adam began to communicate with his parents and change their lives in profound and beautiful ways even before he was born. Martha and John Beck were high-achieving Harvard academics who found out that Martha was pregnant with a child with Down's syndrome. Most people in their academic and medical community urged them to abort. But independently of one another, each parent began experiencing grace-filled paranormal episodes related to their unborn son, who each came to know as "Adam." Many lives have been transformed by this one majestic soul and Martha's sharing of their experiences through her book. And there are many such stories. Tracie Carlos shares similarly moving inspiration in her book *Connor's Gift: Embracing Autism in This New Age.*

What about a baby with a brain tumor or a school child sickened after eating hamburger that turns out to be tainted by a pathogenic strain of normally friendly *E. coli*? How could they be co-creating devastating illness? What about other innocent people who suffer, such as those displaced by wars, children injured by land mines, and those affected by even more unfathomable atrocities? I do not pretend to have specific answers to each of these complex issues. Humanity has long struggled with questions about the suffering of innocents. As I contemplate these questions I have found comfort and peace in responses that link me with my heart.

I understand that I cannot figure it out with my logical mind. The mind is a small, limited part of the infinite all that is. Another Max Planck quote sums this up. Though in his whole quote he is referring to science and not the logical mind, I believe the same applies: "Science cannot solve the ultimate mystery of nature. And that is because, in the last analysis, we ourselves are part of nature and therefore part of the mystery that we are trying to solve."[2] From my limited mind, I do feel distress when I contemplate these questions trying to find understanding. The familiar and depressing feeling of powerlessness sets in. When I feel my way toward a bigger picture, instead of trying to reason my way to it, I notice that focusing on the evolution of tragedies and atrocities always feels terrible. It is like my patients who are still focusing on what they want to let go of. My focus on things that make me feel powerless and despairing glues me to the problems and blinds me to the solutions and peace available. Whenever I get to that spot, my only choice, if I want to feel better, is to know that my true empowerment is to let go and return to my peaceful center. I cannot be part of a solution if I am still mired in the problem. So I breathe and relax, breathe and let go—return to the center of well-being inside me. Return to the me who is constant and unchanged. I contrast my feelings of powerlessness in limitation with knowledge of the Golden World, and even the Silver World. I know that we are unlimited, eternal, and there is a bigger picture. In that bigger picture, nothing is broken. Each person who I see as suffering is actually whole, eternal, and divine. Each is love. Each is "I." I can even rest, nourish myself, and swim in that bigger picture. From that place I have different insights about the world and her woes.

Of course, I do not have to like things that are undesired, whether they are in the arena of health, health care, politics, or social institutions. When I hear of the plight of people affected by tragedies, I have a strong desire for well-being. When I hear about the devastating effects of wars on humans, animals, and the Earth itself, I have a strong desire for peace, and for myself to be a part of creating greater peace. When I learn of devastating health problems, I want to see and know real health, real thriving, greater than anything we have previously experienced upon this planet. I want this personally and for others. I want to be of assistance in creating this flourishing health. From a place of inner peace, I understand that somehow the suffering of innocents is in service of a great good. From a soul level or expanded perspective, they are agreeing to play a part, even though their conscious mind and the minds of their loved ones are usually not aware of this. They are creating more joy, more balance, more love. They want to create greater peace, greater health, greater thriving.

I believe that sometimes there is a bigger message in these seemingly devastating situations that tells us about what we as a society are offering vibrationally. As communities and cultures we offer mixed signals. We are not whole-hearted. Collectively we have accepted compromises that are dehumanizing. We have ceased noticing our discomfort about many cultural and societal norms. As large groups, we have ignored our feelings of dis-ease. Might it then be that some of those suffering souls who are very precious to us offer a loud and clear image of our disconnection? I believe, as I explain below, that often those we see as suffering innocents like small children and newborns are really great teachers of compassion, wholeness, and harmony.

How might this viewpoint change our response to a situation? Consider an unfortunately common scenario. E. coli is normally a healthy bacterium of the gastrointestinal tract. It has many jobs in its cooperative role in our intestinal health. Among them, E. coli manufactures vitamin K2 that is essential for healthy bone metabolism. It also prevents imbalanced and harmful bacteria from lodging in our gut.

Recently, however, there have been numerous outbreaks of "pathogenic life-threatening" strains of E. coli 0157-H7.[3,4] These have been found in meat, particularly hamburgers served predominantly at some fast-food restaurants, but these same bacteria have also been found in meat sold through grocery stores and in hamburger served in schools to children. The unifying factor in all of these meats is that they were cheap, raised industrially, and processed in a mechanized system at huge factories. Lots of meat from lots of sources was mixed together. It was impossible to determine if one giant producer's meat was tainted or if many were, or if the pathogenic E. coli originated at the slaughterhouse. All that we are sure of is that by the time the products departed from the distribution point, the pathogenic bacteria were spread throughout hundreds of thousands of pounds of meat and disseminated widely around the United States.[5]

What could the messages to and from broader consciousness be in this instance? When people sicken from eating these burgers, what might the bacteria and those who have succumbed to illness be demonstrating? Looking at this more deeply, we see there are many areas of potential imbalance. Does the system of delivering meat to the school, store, or restaurant honor life? What about the way the animal was raised? What about how it was slaughtered? We have all been exposed to information about industrial agricultural practices and slaughterhouses that have recently and rapidly become the "conventional" model. In fact, there is nothing "conventional" about this system. Many of us have felt uneasiness about the treatment of animals throughout this industrial system, similar to the disquiet that we experience when we ourselves are cogs in a workforce machine or routed through a mechanized disease-management system.

Cattle are ruminant animals. They are vegetarians who predominantly eat grass, and perhaps a bit of fruit and leaves. They have a second stomach, the rumen, which allows them to digest cellulose in vegetation when they chew their cud. In nature cattle live outdoors, sheltered by trees in inclement weather. But in industrial agriculture, cattle live in cramped buildings and are fed foods unnatural to them including grains, chicken manure, and animal parts (including parts from other dead cattle). Grains like corn may seem innocent but they cannot be digested in the rumen. They give the cattle acid stomach. Plus, most feed-corn is now genetically modified, a further potential hazard. And cattle are vegetarians in nature, so feeding them parts of other cows and chicken manure is truly deranged.

Commercial chicken and eggs are produced under similar circumstances. Chickens are birds. In nature they fly short distances, they roost, and they like to peck in yards. Like all natural animals they live outdoors. Outdoors, they perform chicken-like activities such as eating insects, preening, and taking dirt baths. Compare this to the condition of factory-farmed chickens who live in cages stacked six high. Those chickens never walk on earth. Some of them do not touch the ground for their entire lives. Their beaks are cut off because in such close quarters they become aggressive and attack one another through the wires. They eat food that is not natural for them, and they cannot preen and clean themselves. Chickens in the lower cages become matted with feces from chickens stacked above them. In 2010 in the United States there occurred the most massive recall of eggs ever recorded. A staggering five hundred million eggs were "contaminated" with the bacteria salmonella.[6]

How do we feel about this? The bigger picture reflects something about our disquiet as a society in regard to the ways animals raised for our nourishment are treated. Do you remember our premise of interconnectedness? Some part of us is aware of the lives of these animals. Some part of us, our divinity, *is* these animals. Humans have had a cooperative relationship with certain animals since the dawn of civilization. In this relationship there is a sacred trust, with an unspoken agreement underlying it: I will care for you, and you will live a life of dignity, expressing your animal nature. At the end of this you will nourish me as others—plants, insects, and animals—have nourished you. When I die, I will nourish them, and all this will repeat, each of us expressing our divine natures, in an eternal wheel.

Animals in factory farms do not get to express much of their essential nature. These are more like animal concentration camps, and living in these conditions, animals sicken. Being sick adversely affects the chemical composition of the animal's flesh that we will later consume. The damaged meat becomes a more favorable environment for the flourishing of certain "pathologic" bacteria. When unhealthy animals give out the "come and get me" message, bacteria lovingly respond. These bacteria get distributed in the meat that is produced. They are disseminated widely as meat from multiple sources is mixed together at gargantuan distribution facilities.[7]

The system of balance is broken. Inspectors are bribed to ignore ill cattle at the slaughterhouse, and producers do as much as they can to prop up diseased cattle and make them appear well enough to pass inspection. Standards for chickens and eggs are low, serving high-volume corporate farming interests rather than chickens and eaters. The old system of accountability has broken down, where people who produced food knew the people who consumed it, where they looked each other squarely in the eye and inquired about the health of their children. The "modern" system that has so swiftly replaced it lacks accountability and humanity. No wonder there is dis-ease in the current situation.

In a sacred trust, this situation is deeply out of balance. There is dis-ease, of course, because we all know at some level what is occurring. We *are* the chickens. We *are* the cattle. There is dis-ease because we are not comfortable with the situation, despite our rationalizations. People have harmoniously raised and eaten chickens for thousands of years. Most of those cows and chickens would not have had the opportunity to be born and have their physical lives if they were not destined to be producers of our eggs or food for our plates. But never before have cattle and chickens not been able to express their chicken-ness or their cattle-ness.

Providing deplorable conditions for any being that nourishes us degrades us as well, be it fields of vegetables doused with pesticides or pigs raised in high-rises filled with manure cesspools. It furthers the separation between our spiritual nature and us. It is out of balance, and we know it.

But even with this system, not everyone succumbs to illness. Societally, we understandably cringe when we see that it is the young and the "innocent" who seem most affected. This is often hardest for us to look at because it is those who we see as the most tender who are often the most vulnerable: the young, the elderly, the weak. But we are eternal beings, and there really is no death, only a changing of our energetic form. Might it be that some of those we most cherish, such as small children, decide from a greater soul perspective to be both the image of the imbalance and a directional arrow pointing toward the rebalancing that is needed? Of course, I do not believe the ones who sicken are making this choice from their limited physical-experience perspective. A gravely ill two-year-old does not think she is trying to make a point. Instead, I believe it is a soul-level decision, and the very young and very old who succumb do choose, but not from their physically focused mind. Rather they choose from their eternal nature and from their willingness to carry us all toward greater good and greater love.

Children are closer to their essential nature, closer to the unspoken knowledge that we are all one. Children are closer to the wisdom that we are all spiritual masters mirroring one another for greater love and joy. Young children seem more aware of their divine eternal nature, nearer to the knowledge that there is no real death, just transformation. From the enlightened perspective of their soul, perhaps children who sicken in these new epidemics are cooperative players in bringing awareness, and they are harbingers of change. They certainly do get our attention. Of course, I have no external proof that my concept is correct. I am perhaps trying to understand something the rational mind is incapable of understanding. But in my heart, this line of thought is comforting and peaceful. There, I acknowledge the existence of meaning, dignity, and wholeness. The fear-based response to food-borne bacterial epidemics is to do more killing. We might irradiate the food, or sterilize it with ultra-pasteurization. We might heap a lot of regulation upon industrial food producers, hoping they will earnestly comply. But food is devitalized and chemically altered by measures like irradiation and ultra-pasteurization. Plus, in acting from fear, we miss the message that calls us back to balance, respect, and harmony. As I learned with my sinus infection, when we miss the message, the next one is louder. Every step we take in the direction of fear-based action disconnects us more and more from our spiritual nature. Instead, what is needed is an understanding of what is imbalanced, and a correction of the whole to restore balance.

I believe the industrial models of food supply and health care are merely blips on the screen of human existence. I believe that putting low cost above real nourishment or real health are indicators of a deep disregard for ourselves. In his book *In Defense of Food*, Michael Pollan points out that in 1960 we spent close to eighteen percent of our income on food and five percent on "health care." For years those numbers have been reversing. We now spend just under ten percent of our income on food while health care costs have more than tripled to sixteen percent of our income, and disease "management" costs are climbing. We have copious cheap, poor-quality food, and triple the health care costs. So ask yourself, do you deserve healthy food? Do you deserve to feel comfortable about the treatment of animals and vegetables that you will eat? Do you want to feel good about the way food is raised and produced?

We can make a big difference with our personal choices and an even greater impact through our shift of focus. We do not need to say no to a broken system—we will benefit by saying yes to ourselves. We can say to ourselves, yes, I can eat more foods raised in a system with integrity. Yes, I can make decisions about my body and my health-care choices from a centered, loving place. Yes, I can be whole-hearted in my choices. Yes, I acknowledge that life is sacred, and that to live a physical life I must eat, and to eat I must take life—whether that is plant, bacteria, fungus, or animal. But I choose to participate in a system that honors the web of life, a grand cooperative play where each can express its divine nature. I choose to feel whole-hearted and at peace with nourishment. I choose to feel delight in my miraculous body. I choose to pay attention to how I feel about my choices and to strive to make choices that feel consistent with the best of me. I can make these choices about my food supply and I can make them about my health care. I can listen to my body. I can understand that my body is not betraying me when I am ill but rather reflecting my-self to me. When a societal system is ill, some segment of us, one that we care about—like we personally care about our own bodies, or our children—will give us a message about the imbalance. The greater and more overlooked the imbalance, the louder the message. We can choose to pay attention at any time.

Is misery inevitable in the creation of greater love? Of course it is not. We are at a pivotal juncture in human expansion. The old ways are dying and the new are being born. As we observe suffering caused by pollution, wars, disease, and famine, we hope for a more pacific, easier way to grow in love. We co-create a gentler, more peaceful world through our dreams and desires. Whether we experience it while we live depends upon whether we remain focused upon problems that torture us, or the visionary future that we create when we look toward what we want. We must release dwelling in the misery in order to accept a life embracing wholeness. So notice what you do not like in the world. Notice how wrong it feels. Then let go of focusing upon it. When there is something that feels very wrong, there is its opposite, which feels very right. Let yourself turn your gaze away from the hopelessness and paralysis that seem to accompany every devastating problem. Set your sights toward peace in your inner world and in the outer world. Solutions are born from a fresh, expanded consciousness. What is wanted feels vibrant and alive. Love is the life force, pulsing toward us, resonating through us. There is always something greater that we are expanding toward. You can let it in to heart and mind; you can let mighty waves of peace flow in. With it come the vision, methods, tools, and inspiration to create a better dream of life for all.

TOOLS FOR TRANSFORMATION

When I begin to feel ill, I examine what is going on for me spiritually and emotionally. If there is a microbe involved, I send love to the bacteria, virus, or fungus that is helping me to notice the imbalance. If something else is amiss—a back spasm or a nosebleed—I send love to the cells and tissues involved. I quiet myself and listen inwardly. As I contemplate with this attitude of love, a transformation always occurs. I have learned to trust this process although it was alien to my medical training. With patients who are interested in and asking for this approach, I provide similar coaching. With anything deep, severe, or chronic, I find that the cause is usually some habitual way of being so entrenched that we no longer notice the discomfort it causes. Our physical body amplifies our emotional or spiritual discomfort so we can pay attention. This may be about feeling unsafe in the world, or feeling like we are not good enough or worthy enough or attractive enough. It may be because we see brokenness in the external world instead of wholeness, or that we are fearful.

When you feel ill, it is possible to discuss the concern with the area involved.

1. Center in your heart, perhaps through some of the breathing techniques mentioned previously. Find a place of serenity and calm within yourself.
2. Breathe in through your heart and out to the area of the concern. Then reverse this, breathing in through the area and back to the heart. Do this several times.
3. Send love to the area. Let it know that you understand there is a message and ask for gentle assistance in interpreting it.
4. Notice if any impressions, thoughts, insights, or images come to you. You must relax for them to come. If you stay in the mode of asking the question, you cannot hear an answer. So just breathe and relax, letting your mind be clear of thoughts and questions.
5. If no answers come right away, don't worry. The energetic connection has been opened and in time you will have greater clarity. Pay attention to your dreams and continue to try the exchange on other days. Take a walk in nature!

It is also possible to discuss what you would like with the bacteria, virus, or fungus.

Again, try this tool from a quiet or meditative frame of mind and heart:

1. Acknowledge their right to exist, and their important place in the balance of life.
2. Explain what symptoms you are having and how you would like to feel. If they would like a place to grow and replicate in you while you remain healthy, let them know that is fine, if you feel it is okay.

All microbes, in my experience, are able to happily cooperate when we communicate consciousness to consciousness.

—CHAPTER ELEVEN—

Cooperation/Community: Fungi

SOIL CAN BE SEEN AS both an enormous single living organism and as an interrelated community. There are innumerable inextricably intertwined participants in a healthy soil neighborhood including bacteria, insects, fungi, mosses, lichens, viruses, and animals. Small animals aerate soil with their burrows, providing runnels for water to flow. Larger animals contribute to the soil daily by depositing their waste products. Animals nourish the soil even in death as their bodies, bones, and blood decompose to contribute to the web of life. Blood, in small amounts, is especially nutritious to soil, so perhaps that is why, in folklore, there are numerous tales of flowers springing up where blood has been spilled.

Thriving soil is laced with a fungus called mycorrhiza that supports the roots of most plants, including trees. Mycorrhizae form a mycelium, a single lacy mesh of underground plant life. Individually, mycelial organisms are miniscule and threadlike; in one cubic inch of healthy soil there can be up to eight miles of microscopic mycorrhizal filaments and several thousand species of fungus. But as a community, mycorrhizae constitute the largest organisms living on the planet and are essential for healthy soil. Some individual mycorrhizal organism communities are known to extend for miles.[1] These fungi are cooperative with the many plants they support, and neither flourishes without the other. Mycorrhizae have many gifts to offer other plants since they structure and stabilize the soil, forming an underground network through which above-ground plants weave their roots. Tree roots intertwine with the mycorrhizal mycelial tissue, forming a dense branching pattern beneficial for both species. The mycorrhizae hold moisture near the plant's roots, allowing them to thrive even when there is relative drought or poor soil conditions.

Mycorrhizae also assist in the exchange of nutrients, especially phosphorus, at the roots of many plants. In turn, plants and trees supply the mycorrhizae with metabolic products that nourish and support them, such as the carbohydrates glucose and sucrose. The mycorrhizal fungi eat dead plant tissues and discarded materials that are no longer needed. They decompose these, acting as mini compost piles at the base of each root, by recycling nutrients into their own healthy tissue and then making them available for the plant or tree to utilize again. Mycorrhizae contribute greatly to bio-diversity in plants, helping support a healthy balance of organisms in the soil community. Earthworms are also essential for maintaining and aerating healthy soil, composting organic debris and freeing it to nourish new life. Charles Darwin's final but least famous book was entirely about earthworms and their essential role in the health of the soil.

Approximately ninety-five percent of plant species live in com-munity with mycorrhizae and earthworms. Pesticides, herbicides, and fungicides sprayed on crops, and terminator genes from genetically modified organisms, can disrupt and kill both mycorrhizae and earth-worms. These staples of modern "conventional" agriculture weaken the very structure of the soil. Where mycorrhizae and earthworms are absent or scarce, above-ground plant communities are undermined. They grow debilitated, and in this condition (just like humans in a similar state) plants are much more susceptible to "disease."

All communities and ecosystems include members that work with decay, waste, and even scavenging. When plants are devitalized, as they are from the destruction of their mycorrhizal companions, they emit pheromones like those I discussed earlier—the chemical messag-es that attract scavengers. Parasitic nematodes, ancillary participants in the process of decomposition, begin to flourish. Parasitic nema-todes, viruses, and insects are drawn to depleted plant communities by the messages emitted by the plants themselves.

The view of industrial agriculture is that these recycling organisms are baneful, unwanted pests. The parasitic nematodes, however, are just doing their job, finding a niche, and supporting their communities in the absence of other thriving soil organisms, including normal organisms of decomposition. Nematodes contribute to balance and are found in small numbers in healthy soil. Nematodes are the undertakers of the soil community. We need undertakers; they are a necessary and respected segment of the population. Still, we would not desire a situation where our need for undertakers was as plentiful as our need for childcare workers or restaurant personnel. This would indicate that a serious imbalance is occurring, with more people requiring burial and fewer needing baby-tending or delicious food.

"Pests" are just doing what they do naturally: responding to the lack of health and vitality in the plants themselves and participating in recycling. It does not matter to them if these particular vegetables are what were recently planted on a given farm and the farmer has a large loan leveraged against the presumed profits from the harvest. Just like our bodies do not know the difference between the stress of malnutrition due to anorexia nervosa and the stress of malnutrition due to famine, nature in her adaptive patterns cannot tell the difference between plants not thriving because their synergistic mycorrhizal mycelia family has been destroyed by pesticides and herbicides, and sickness caused by some other factor like drought. In all these cases the devitalized plants emit the chemical and vibrational message, "I am sick, I am weak, it is time for those of you who can thrive in this situation to come and dine, recycling the elements of my body for new life."

A large part of the imbalance of industrial agriculture is caused by its exclusive reliance upon monocultures—farming systems where only one species is planted or encouraged to flourish. Think of the hundreds of miles of corn and soybean fields that are the Great Plains today. Almost every other living thing is considered a pest, and other plants are "weeds." There are few small foraging animals and insects, largely limited to ones the farmer might think of as "pests." Since there is only one food to eat, the species that prefer exactly what the farmer has planted are the only ones who will survive in any number. In naturally occurring ecosystems there are no monocultures.

Until very recently, the Great Plains were diverse prairie ecosystems, home to tens of thousands of species above and below the soil. The thick rich soil of the Great Plains was built over thousands of years. It can take up to five hundred years for nature to build one inch of topsoil. About six inches of topsoil are required for good crop production. The primarily hunter/gatherer dietary choices and lifestyle of plains-dwelling Native Americans encouraged the diversity that supported the growth of magnificent topsoil. Native American cultures see humans as stewards of the land. They had many different religions, but all of them acknowledged interconnectedness among people, land, and nature. The soil built richly during their tenure, as it had in the ages before humans inhabited North America. The health of Native American people also thrived. European explorers remarked over and over about the vigor, stamina, clear skin, and fine straight teeth of the populations they encountered here.

Today, the formerly thick topsoil layer, built cooperatively over thousands of years, has been reduced dramatically in a mere century. Estimates indicate that the thickness of the topsoil of much of the arable land of the Great Plains has dipped from twelve inches to just four inches in the last forty years alone.[2] In a 1937 letter to State Governors advocating a uniform soil conservation law, President Theodore Roosevelt said, "The nation that destroys its soil, destroys itself." Yet in the years since he wrote those prescient words, the United States has seen its soil rapidly eroded, degraded, and lost, largely through government subsidization of unsustainable industrial agriculture practices.

Monoculture-dependent industrial agriculture is a soil-destroying aberration deeply out of balance with the natural world. With this understanding, we can realize that agricultural "pests" and disease-causing super-bugs are actually our friends within a bigger picture. Dividing the world into organisms that we like and organisms we do not like (based on how it benefits a few of us in the short term), without consideration for the interrelatedness of all life or future generations, is unfortunately myopic. Agribusinesses and frightened farmers are afraid the bugs will destroy this year's crop, so they use pesticides and herbicides on fields that ruin the health of the soil. Newly "conventional" farming practices push the soil to extreme production by adding just a few nutrients—nitrogen, phosphorus, and potassium—into a diverse and complex system. All the other minerals are depleted by growing plants but not replenished. Then we are shocked after a few years that our soil health is poor and our crops are not thriving. Our children exhibit deficiencies that show up in a myriad of new ailments, because food produced in this manner is of poor quality and lacks essential minerals. Advertising takes over, attempting to brainwash people into believing that denuded, empty foods are "wholesome."

For an eye-opening experience, do a Web search to compare levels of essential minerals like calcium, magnesium, manganese, selenium, and zinc in common foods with their former levels of fifty or a hundred years ago. Newly "conventional" foods have only a small fraction of these essential building blocks of health. As a society we make unwise choices by looking at just the next one or two seasons, or the next one or two fiscal cycles, without regard for the wisdom of the whole and without consultation with our hearts.

The National Academy of Sciences characterizes the density of fertile soil by the amount of carbon present. Carbon is found in various plant, insect, and animal tissues. After water, which is hydrogen and oxygen, carbon is the most plentiful element in our bodies. Carbon in the soil is good for the health of almost all life on Earth, as the vast majority of living organisms are carbon-based. Soil carbon is the single largest reservoir of the element. Its level in the soil is an essential factor in understanding climate change.

The bodies of ancient plants and animals along with geothermal pressure from the Earth produced petroleum millions of years ago. These forces, over time, created a large reserve of carbon that was held deep in the planet's crust. The soil and living beings form another large pool. Relatively little carbon is atmospheric, and the level of carbon in the air (as well as other gases) relates to what is popularly called "the greenhouse effect." Some atmospheric carbon is essential for terrestrial life; it is taken in by plants during photosynthesis and converted into organic matter. But the amount of atmospheric carbon required by plants can be provided by animal respiration alone. Humans and other animals exhale carbon as carbon dioxide when we breathe, returning carbon to the atmosphere. Prior to the age of petroleum products and industrial agriculture, the amount of carbon absorbed by plants balanced the amount of carbon exhaled by animals and insects. Today, the ancient reserves of carbon once stored deep in the earth as petroleum and coal, as well as significant amounts of the carbon reservoir in soil,[3] have been released into the atmosphere through combustion and other metabolic processes like digestion and gassification. In simple terms, excess carbon in the atmosphere instead of in the earth is what many researchers believe causes climate change—both warming and cooling.

Many studies have evaluated how much carbon has been lost from soils secondary to erosive processes caused by contemporary agriculture. The results are disturbing. With deep soil tillage by large machines, carbon is rapidly shifted to the atmosphere, decreasing the thickness of topsoil. The resulting increase in atmospheric temperatures hastens the carbon loss and soil erosion. Losses are significant enough that they can be tracked annually.[4]

It is possible, and perhaps not even very difficult, to reverse erosion and possibly global warming, while building soil fertility and topsoil.

Cooperation with nature is the answer, entailing a different model of agriculture than the one offered to us by multinational corporations. There are many encouraging models indicating that we could sink large volumes of carbon back into the soil relatively quickly, benefiting soil fertility, species diversity, and the overall health of humanity and other life. The Soil Association, a British charity dedicated to "campaigning for planet-friendly food and farming,"[5] estimates that if all British agriculture were shifted to organic cultivation, 32 million tons of carbon would be removed from the atmosphere annually. This is equivalent to one million fewer cars on the road, from British farms alone.[6]

Joel Salatin is a popular speaker and Virginia farmer. He calls himself a grass farmer because he practices a type of agriculture that supports diverse communities of grasses that animals rotationally graze upon. He also calls himself an earthworm farmer. His methods rely on mimicry of nature to build soil fertility, rapidly increase topsoil, and sink carbon into the earth. He grows some organic crops rotationally, as well as raising abundant healthy livestock on the rich soil he has cultivated on his farm. Salatin's parents bought their tract of land in 1961. The parcel was cheap because it was eroded and "worn out." Instead of following the then-popular industrial practices, the Salatins chose to use nature as their teacher. They planted trees and grasses, built huge compost piles, and encouraged wildlife diversity through maintaining riparian areas near cropped fields. They rotated grazing animals daily to support the health of the grasses that nourish these animals. They tilled sparingly. The Salatins learned from the wisdom of generations of traditional farmers. They found that small-scale farming in cooperation with nature enriches and builds soil, which, in turn, nourishes humans and other life. Salatin calls his prosperous and thriving farm "Polyface Farm,"[7] indicating both the biodiversity and the multiple farm products that he and his family raise.

This type of agriculture is only feasible for small and mid-size farms. Though profitable, it is labor-intensive and cannot be practiced on a large scale. It is perfect for families and communities. There are no monocultures in this model. Instead, resilience-building diversity is encouraged. Industry argues that this model is inefficient, but the great preponderance of evidence indicates that this natural model is far more efficient than large agribusiness. In April 2008, the final report of the United Nations International Assessment of Agricultural Knowledge, Science and Technology for Development (IAASTD) was published. The document represents the work of four hundred scientists worldwide, and it indicts industrial farming as energy-draining and toxic.[8] The paper, endorsed by sixty countries including the UK and most European nations but not the United States, calls for a radical shift in basic farming practices to address hunger, social inequity, environmental degradation, and cost of food production. The report encourages small-scale agriculture[9] and organic and ecological cultivation as we move forward.

With more permaculture and organic small-scale agriculture, more higher-quality food is produced from each acre. Topsoil is built up and enhanced soil fertility sinks atmospheric carbon into thick humus. Many more jobs supplying living wages are created, and biodiversity thrives. Polyculture small-scale farming is ideal for the planet, other species, and humanity. It builds local communities and economies.

Several scholars have analyzed the impact of shifting agriculture to widespread polyculture grass-based farming. The projections from these models are astounding. If adopted widely, polyculture grass farming theoretically could reverse the greenhouse effect from carbon emissions causing current climate change in as little as ten years.[10] Soil fertility and topsoil quantity would improve dramatically, and food nutrient quality would rise. This would be a big shift in our farming practices and our social systems.

Why don't we hear anything about this simple solution in the media or from government? For one, we would have to stop the war against nature, and acknowledge that nature is wise. The premises of society tend to lean toward the opinions of powerful vested interests. The influence and profits of large industries decline as many more small independent farms and self-reliant communities flourish.

Cooperation with nature can solve many other perplexing contemporary problems. Working with mycelia and mushrooms, for example, we can clean up toxic oil spills. Mushroom wizard Paul Stamets does just that. Basing his research upon a model that mimics nature, he developed methods of growing mushrooms for bioremediation (a.k.a. toxic clean-up). These fungi are capable of restoring the purity of polluted water, rapidly clearing oil spills, and decontaminating wastes.[11] The fungi produce healthy soil, compost, and humus. Benign algae colonies can also be grown that consume pollutants in water, harmlessly clarifying it and returning it to purity.

I would venture to say that looking to nature and offering cooperation and respect could solve all our current imbalances rapidly and efficiently. Some forests require fire as part of a natural cycle to support new life. Certain seeds cannot germinate unless they are scorched by fire. When small fires are not allowed to burn, eventually debris builds up on the forest floor and huge devastating fires result. Through painful experience, the National Forest Service personnel now understand this and practice controlled burns in many forests they manage.

Floodplains experience floods. Instead of trying to build a large metropolis upon them and making lots of dams to hold back the normal flow of water, there is a burgeoning acknowledgement that these are not the ideal locations for large cities. Insurers, including the federal government, are encouraging development elsewhere by refusing to provide flood insurance for structures built in areas that will inevitably flood.

In ecology there is a progression of species in any system. I view contemporary agriculture as one short-lived species in a long chain of diversity. By taking monocultures to the extreme, corporations have done us a favor. They have rapidly shown to us the many ways that a model that disregards or tries to subdue nature is fundamentally flawed and unsustainable. Life in any ecosystem is a study in cooperation and balance. By studying, mimicking, and delicately enhancing the nuances of nature we learn to thrive.

Similarly, any physical illness provides a wealth of metaphorical information to the person or community that is affected. One way to approach health problems is to examine them through the lens of nature. Look for what healthy role the disease-causing agent has in nature. In this light, we can learn a lot from fungus. Health issues relating to overgrowth of fungi are commonplace in a family-practice setting. I find them fascinating, as they provide a rich trove of symbolic wisdom to the inquisitive patient.

As we have seen, fungus is a communal organism much like ants are communal insects. They grow in vast cooperative networks, especially in dark, damp places like the soil. They spread in a web-like manner through underground filamentous projections. Most of the life of terrestrial fungus is subterranean. Above-ground mushrooms and other fruiting bodies of fungus are a minute fraction of their mass.

In humans, the soil in which fungus embeds is human tissue. As in the Earth's soil, fungi grow well in stagnant areas with persistent dampness. On the planet's surface, fungi have many important roles. They enliven stagnation and clear it, getting things moving again, as demonstrated by the example of stagnant water purification via fungus-catalyzed bioremediation.

In Chinese medicine as well, dampness is associated with stagnation. Excessive dampness in the digestive tract results in bloating, heaviness, fullness, and murkiness that can also express as cloudy thought, rumination, cysts or tumors, and in severe cases, insanity. Dampness interferes with the conversion of food nutrients to energy, bone, blood, and thought. Dampness in the lungs leads to phlegm, cough, shortness of breath, infections, and anxiety. Once dampness is prevalent in the system, it can be slow to transform.

Likewise, once fungus is established, it can be difficult to clear up without significant changes in behavior and attitude. Fungi, like humans, are complex multicellular organisms. The pharmaceutical model of killing fungus is problematic because the things that kill "them" kill "us" too. Many antifungal drugs are toxic, especially to the liver, our main organ of detoxification. Fungi interlace themselves through our tissues and do not give up easily. Fungal die-off rapidly releases many products of stagnation back into our system that the fungi had been slowly transforming.

Fungi bind to heavy metals, forming fungal-metal complexes. This is well known in the mining industry. Mining operations frequently inject fungus into deep veins of ore to bring it to the surface. If a person has a heavy load of fungus in their system, I have learned to look for the presence of heavy metals. The individual may think the fungus is "the problem" but, in actuality, the fungus may be protecting them from the much more alarming effects of excessive toxic metals like mercury.

Therefore many people with yeast overgrowth syndrome prefer to remain on a milder program of protracted dietary restrictions, gentle detoxification, and shifting of thoughts and beliefs. (Yeasts like *Candida albicans* are types of fungi commonly associated with humans.) This allows the excess fungus to slowly clear as their body gradually eliminates bound metals and toxins, and allows time for the murkiness in their thoughts and emotional overwhelm to settle and clarify as well.

Any infection has a lot to teach us about ourselves. Emotionally and spiritually, fungus present in the body leads people metaphorically to deep, stagnant issues. Filaments of these issues touch and affect many areas of life. Fungal infections often illuminate core issues, longstanding and deeply held beliefs, and protracted dysfunctional patterns of action that affect the individual broadly.

Fungus is never simple, though sometimes it is not particularly dangerous. For example, a common skin fungus is *Tinea versicolor,* a flat, patchy fungus that grows most often on the back and chest. It is notoriously difficult to eradicate but is more of a nuisance and cosmetically unappealing problem than a serious health concern. It is communicable, but not easily. One patient I know has it, but his wife does not. She has not contracted it so far during the seven years of their marriage. They have produced two lovely children, so there is evidence that there has been an exchange of sweat, and skin-to-skin contact.

We can appreciate the fungus and what it offers. Patients often find that the emotional and spiritual issues related to fungus are interwoven in their lives, affecting many ways of being, just as fungus interweaves in tissue. When I have patients with a fungal overgrowth, I encourage them to look for deep-seated and possibly stagnant issues that entangle many areas of their life.

Take, for example, a digestive fungal overgrowth. I encourage patients with this condition to consider looking at ways they are not digesting their life. Examining their words to themselves and their basic behaviors is often fruitful and illuminating.

I have one patient, "Janet," who had a persistent and severe fungal overgrowth in her digestive tract, confirmed by stool tests. She could not tolerate any sweet foods. Even raw carrots or butternut squash triggered symptoms of anal itching, terrible bloating, and skin rash. When we looked at her life, there was a lot that the fungus was showing her. Her life severely lacked sweetness. She described her husband as aloof yet controlling, belittling and disdainful of her. She had really wanted children. She believes her yeast symptoms began around the time her husband flatly refused to consider more offspring (he had two children with his first wife) and had a vasectomy without consulting her. She "knew" she should leave him but she feared destitution if she divorced. He is wealthy and their pre-nuptial agreement was very restrictive. She also described him as "vindictive."

When we looked deeper we saw that none of these issues was new in her life. She and her husband, who was older and very much like her father, had been married for more than fifteen years. Her mother had been "beaten down" and escaped into quiet alcoholism in her fifties, dying of breast cancer at sixty-two.

This case, although extreme, is not atypical of the deep types of problems that fungi can illuminate and help us clarify. Fungi, infections, and disease processes have wisdom to share with us. They are not "the problem," and thinking of them in that way can derail our healing by preventing us from seeing their gifts.

Many people, led by Dr. Tulio Simoncini in Italy, believe cancer to be a fungus. I have no idea if this theory will prove to be correct, but there are certainly vibrational similarities between the messages of cancer and the messages of fungus. Cancer slowly eats away at us, spreading into tissues through filaments as well as seeding into new tissues through the blood and lymph. Numerous studies have shown that candida (yeast) overgrowth is present in eighty to ninety-five percent of cancer patients.[12] Emotionally, cancer relates to deep, long-standing subterranean issues and internal conflicts that the individual has not been able to clarify. Physically, both cancer and fungus lead to composting of the body, eventually turning tissues back into humus for new life to flourish.

Today Janet is improving. She began psychotherapy and consulted a divorce attorney to better understand her rights. It turns out that her situation is not so bleak as she had imagined, and although she would not be wealthy after a divorce she would be comfortable. She has realized that happiness is the most important thing to her and has been spending more time outdoors by the bay. She got a dog that she loves and who adores her. She carries his picture on her phone. Janet remains careful with her diet and considers the fungus a teacher; she can now eat carrots and an occasional serving of berries without any flare of her symptoms.

As spiritual beings living a physical existence, we have a lot to learn from fungus. We learn about what we have buried, we learn about embedded and deep issues, we learn about interconnection and cooperation. We can learn from any part of nature by befriending it, for we are nature, so we are merely befriending ourselves.

TOOLS FOR TRANSFORMATION

1. There are many refinements available to the basic breathing exercises I have detailed in other chapters. When there is a health issue, including one that is serious or longstanding, try breathing between any affected area and the heart. (Obviously, you are technically breathing in and out through nostrils or mouth; I am speaking of an energetic flow here.)

   Say, for example, that you have a sore knee. You can breathe gently in and out through the heart, or in through the heart and out through the upper abdomen below the breastbone. When you are feeling a sense of calm, then breathe in through your heart, and out through the sore knee. Then breathe in through the knee and out through the heart. Do this a few times. Let the knee (or other affected body part) know that you love it. Feel your appreciation for your body as you breathe in and out.

2. You might also include two other areas in your breathing exercise.

   The crown at the top of the head energetically connects us with the greater whole. You can imagine healing light pouring in through your crown, and flow that light with your out-breath to any place that needs help. This light can be any color that seems soothing and healing, though often people notice green, rose, gold, and violet.

   You can connect your heart, breath, and the affected area with the *ajna* center, also known as the third eye or brow chakra, located in the center of the forehead between the crests of the eyebrows. In Ayurvedic cosmology, this is the seat of intuition. To do this exercise, first center in the heart, breathing in and out. Next, breathe in through the heart and out through the brow, then back in through the brow and out through the heart. Finally, complete the circuit by adding the affected area. Breathe in lightly through the brow, touching the heart energy, then out through the affected area. Then reverse: in through the affected part, touch the heart, out through the brow. Try each of these energy flows a few times.

Engaging our energetic body consciously in these ways, we can access intuitive wisdom that our waking mind normally filters out. We gain valuable insight and deep comfort.

—CHAPTER TWELVE—

Truth: Corporations, Big Pharma, and Me

WHAT IS TRUTH? THIS BURNING question has fueled the work of philosophers for all of recorded history. However, no one has been able to come up with a truth that is absolute and applies to all people, much less one that applies to all life or all of the manifest universe. Truth is not one thing. Of necessity, any discussion of truth follows from our discussion of premises, since truth changes depending on the premises accepted. We have seen that premises are frequently regarded as "truth," until they are discarded for newer or more fashionable beliefs.

Truth, a word that implies objectivity, is subjective. Truth relates to the perspective of the observer. Truth is more of a philosophical ideal than an actual event. Each of us has our individual truth. And for most of us there is heart-truth and there is head-truth. Rationally, we may be persuaded to believe one thing while our heart tells us something quite different. Which is really true? We each have our reasons for deciding upon our personal truths. For example, from a scientific perspective there is tremendous evidence pointing to the truth of various forms of extrasensory perception. Even the most hard-nosed scientist should be persuaded by the preponderance of evidence of multiple studies performed to exacting standards over the last hundred years.

The general public already believes in these phenomena and does not care much about the science supporting it. They ironically accept psi phenomena because of something science shuns: anecdotal evidence. The public believes in ESP because many have experienced it themselves. Others are acquainted with people they know and trust who have had these experiences. You know the type of stories: Uncle John has a knack with anything mechanical—he seems to communicate with engines. Or cousin Marjorie tells you, "I had a bad feeling about the crab dip so I didn't eat it even though I usually love crab dip. Turned out it was tainted and everyone who had some got sick." Or your friend Susan relates that she had a hunch to get off the freeway a few stops early, and she later finds out that there was a major accident up ahead that she might have been caught up in. Stories of hunches and knacks are common. There are more dramatic stories as well—of distance healing, seeing and speaking with people who have died, angels and dead relatives pulling children out of cars after accidents and depositing them uninjured by the roadside, and people who remember past lives in incredible, verifiable detail.

Most scientists, on the other hand, the ones whom the psi researchers presumably care about persuading, staunchly refuse to accept evidence even of the very highest quality. In his book *The Conscious Universe*, Dean Radin, PhD, points out that elite scientists, the ones with the most to lose if psychic phenomena are accepted as "proven," steadfastly refuse to consider the evidence. He notes that seventy percent of the general public believes in the phenomena, but only six percent of top-tier scientists accept them.[1] What is the truth? Truth in this example seems to relate not to "evidence" but to preconceived notions and even bias. The average guy on the street is more open to the evidence than the skeptical scientist who has built a career upon researching the mechanistic model of life.

We see many who lay claim to the truth, but this is usually in the service of some end. The idea of truth seems noble but actually puts us smack into dichotomization. If this is true, then that is false. If this is correct, than that is wrong. So what is the problem? Truths are relative. Truths either form the premises from which conclusions are drawn or are the result of reasoning from selected premises. If, for example, it is true that my God is the one true God, then all of you non-believers are infidels. All of you are wrong. We have seen quite a lot of that reasoning in the last two thousand years, resulting in crusades, holocausts, and cultural genocides. Every one of us has our own precious truth dear to our own heart. My truth may be opposed to your truth.

Culturally in-favor truths will always tend to serve the interests of the powerful, the wealthy, and the victorious. The push toward more globalization as a supposed good is a perfect example of a culturally accepted truth that serves only a small fraction of the population of the planet yet is widely accepted. Is it better for local communities to have a lot of cheap consumer goods from Asia sold at big-box retail conglomerates, while mom-and-pop stores and local producers are driven out of business?

Certain truths are cherished by some cultures. Some truths, like non-acceptance of psi phenomena, are insisted upon as prerequisites for acceptance into the group, or into civil society. In these situations, the concept of truth is all too often applied to keep members in line and discourage dissent. During the worst years of the Khmer Rouge regime in Cambodia, intellectualism was an evil, punishable by death.

What we perceive as truth changes frequently. In past eras physicians believed that bloodletting would cure a patient. They also thought it was unnecessary to wash one's hands while attending a birthing mother and scoffed at the idea of an invisible world of microbes. In the nineteenth century (not so long ago), physicians openly mocked Dr. Ignaz Semmelweis, the Hungarian physician who maintained that merely washing one's hands between attending an autopsy and a delivery would save the lives of countless women. No one could see these so-called organisms, so it was laughable to them that they could be responsible for childbed fever. During the Crimean war, "Sanitationists" who accepted Semmelweis' ideas were considered crackpot "radicals." In each era, the majority of people believed in and accepted "truths" that we now deride.

More recently, in Western nations, women in menopause were routinely put on hormone replacement "therapy." The drug company with the lion's share of the market produces its hormones from the urine of pregnant mares. To produce this wonder drug, pregnant mares are constantly kept in small stalls with catheters inserted that collect all their urine. When the foals are born, they are swiftly killed or sold, so the mare can be re-impregnated and continue her job as a drug factory. When I was in medical school, from 1985 to 1989, we were taught that "science" had demonstrated the truth that women who took these cruelty-full hormones had a lower risk of heart disease and stroke. This was a well-known fact in the mid 1980s. No one questioned the coincidence that the studies demonstrating this advantage were commissioned and paid for by the same pharmaceutical companies that sold the medications. Then in the late 1990s a sharp reversal took place. A rare independent study showed conclusively that women who used these drugs had *higher* rates of heart disease, stroke, and cancer.

In my early twenties, I spent two years in graduate school studying comparative religions. When I chose to enter medicine, a "scientific" field, the parallels between our cultural perception of science and religious belief were not lost on me. Of course, many others have seen that science is the new religion. Thomas Szasz, for example, wrote: "Formerly, when religion was strong and science was weak, men mistook magic for medicine; now, when science is strong and religion weak, men mistake medicine for magic."[2] And like any religion, we are exhorted to believe but not to question the methodologies or the conclusions.

Over the last one hundred years, our society has become enamored with the idea of "scientific truth" as if science itself were an immutable fact like the sun rising each morning. But regarding science it is we who make the observations and call our interpretations of them "laws." Science, at its core, is merely a methodology that humans developed for examination of phenomena. It is formed of our own imperfect belief systems. We decide the parameters, the premises, and the assumptions. We invent the methodologies. We make, and break, the rules. It is ironic, but very human, that we turn around and worship what we ourselves have created. We look at scientific studies and believe in them as if they were eternal truths, even though many of these "truths" last only a few years.

In contemporary society almost all science is driven by profit. We speak of "pure science" as if it were an unassailable ideal understanding separate from human intervention. Yet at the very heart of contemporary science, quantum physics has taught us that we cannot take the observer out of the field of observation. Or, more simply, the mere fact of observing a process changes it and may determine its outcome.

When I was a fifth-grader, my dad, who loved mathematics as I did, gave me Darrell Huff's book *How to Lie with Statistics*. This enduring text was first published in 1954 and remains a classic in the field. It has always been a great source of cautionary amusement to me, as it presents clearly how, without falsifying any data, statistics can be manipulated to imply virtually whatever an author desires. Huff warns readers at the outset, "The secret language of statistics, so appealing in a fact-minded culture, is employed to sensationalize, inflate, confuse, and oversimplify."[3]

For example, "post hoc ergo propter hoc" is a logical fallacy that continues to be employed to imply proven causality when, in fact, none is present. The Latin phrase means literally "after this, therefore because of this." Practically, this implies that if the timing of a second event follows a first one, then the first one caused the second one. It is a fallacy because it relies solely on the temporal sequence of events to prove causality, where generally none exists. So an absurd example of this would be the belief that since ambulances are generally observed at the scene after motor vehicle accidents, they must therefore cause the smash-ups. We see this type of logical fallacy applied constantly in medicine and medical research. The debate about cholesterol is a currently active question that relies upon this fallacy. We observe that cholesterol is found in atherosclerotic plaque. Does this mean it "causes" the plaque? Possibly, but there are many other equally plausible interpretations, including the possibility that cholesterol is a repair molecule mopping up damage done by something else, like inflammation. Whenever you find the word "associated" appearing in a discussion of a medical study, be aware that many times what has been associated is merely the timing of two potentially unrelated events.

A related fallacy is "cum hoc ergo propter hoc," or "with this, therefore because of this." Here it is assumed that two events occurring together are related. However, we learn in basic statistics that correlation does not imply causation. Again, consider the example of hormone replacement therapy (HRT). It was initially noted that women who used HRT had fewer heart attacks than the general population. In this case, the fallacy was the assumption that the HRT caused the decrease in heart attacks. Eventually, though, a study was done showing that the drugs actually *increased* heart attacks. The previous assumption was traced to the fact that women who used (and could afford) HRT tended to be from higher socio-economic backgrounds, and as a group they had better nutrition and exercised more than the general population. When this group was studied separately with and without the drugs, it was observed that those *off* the drugs clearly had fewer heart attacks.

It would be comforting to believe that physicians, who have advanced degrees, would not be susceptible to basic logical fallacies. Comforting, but unfortunately untrue. Medical training does not include even a basic course in logic, and sadly, most doctors are easily swayed by logical fallacies such as these demonstrated above. Many studies are reported as associations, as if association really means anything definitive about causation.

Now, if I were a chemical manufacturer, a pharmaceutical company, or a biotech firm, it is understandable that I would have some investment, both financially and emotionally, in the results of scientific exploration in areas of investigation related to my products. Today we have a particularly deplorable situation where "the foxes" do the research, with no obligation to publish data showing negative consequences for "the hens." In medicine today, especially in the United States, we also have a situation where the governmental regulatory agencies, originally mandated to serve in roles of impartial oversight, are now filled with paid consultants and cronies of the industries they oversee. Scandal after scandal has shown us that manufacturers "knew" of problems, and negative results were "buried," that regulatory agencies were silenced or bought off, or complicit because their offices were filled by industry representatives. We then learn, if we are paying attention, that doctors get most of their information about drugs from drug company representatives. Unfortunately, the identical "fox guarding the henhouse" situation exists in other governmental agencies as well. The USDA, for example, is filled with representatives of agribusiness. The network of corporate influence in our society and the "scientific truths" they promote are staggering.

Regarding drug interaction, we naively believe that these potentially problematic combinations are studied, but by whom? Drug companies do most of the studies. Multiple drugs are seldom studied in combination, even if they are routinely prescribed in combinations. Physician advisors on the drug company payroll endorse them.

Over and over again we see "truth" in medicine or nutrition or agriculture defined by biased groups. One of my close childhood friends became a psychiatrist. She was well respected in her region and told me how she would often be invited to lunch meetings at posh restaurants as a member of this or that drug company's "advisory panel." At these "committee meetings," doctors would have a great lunch and chat amongst themselves. Then, briefly, the pharmaceutical company employees would detail their drug-du-jour, and the hand-picked group of physicians attending would agree to endorse it. At the end of the lunch, every "advisor" who endorsed, which was pretty much every physician there, would be handed a check for $1,000, $1,500, or even $2,000. She explained that being on an advisory panel meant lending her good name and reputation and listening to an "educational" spiel. She had no obligation to actually give advice or even report positive or negative findings once she was prescribing the drugs. Invitations to future lucrative lunches were dependent upon the numbers of prescriptions written for the new drugs. These prescriptions were tracked through national corporate pharmacy chains. My friend confided in me that she was deeply conflicted about this. She attended such advisory committee meetings frequently, often every couple of weeks, as they substantially enhanced her income, which helped her family. Still, she felt her position was unethical and that the new drugs were often no better, and sometimes much worse, than the existing medications.

Truth and facts are often used synonymously. They are similar. But fact, like truth, is another tricky word. "Fact" implies objectivity but remains subjective. We look at facts to establish the truth. I thought about this one morning as I ate my breakfast, loosely gazing at the nutrition "facts" on my yogurt container. I thought, what is factual about this? Isn't this a perspective? Who sets nutrition policy in the United States and what are their objectives? What other nutrition "facts" are not reported? Why are these particular nutrients presented and not others? Who determines the RDAs for them and why?

The contrast between the media's treatment of psi research and nutrition science is informative. Psi research is belittled by calling it a "pseudoscience." This reflects observer/reporter bias because often psi research is among the most scientifically rigorous type of experimentation performed. Meanwhile, shoddily done nutrition research gets called "fact" while it is more aptly pseudoscience. Even prominent nutritionists acknowledge that research in this field is woefully inadequate.

The root of the word "fact" is the Latin *factum*, meaning "something done," which further derives from the Latin verb *facere*, meaning "to make." Recalling the levels of interpretation of texts that I discussed earlier, we see that a hint, or *remez*, is found in the root of the word "fact." These roots imply that fact is a creation. The *World English Dictionary Online* has many definitions of fact. These include:

1. An event or thing known to have happened or existed
2. A truth verifiable from experience or observation
3. A piece of information: get me all the facts of this case
4. (Often plural) law: an actual event, happening, etc., as distinguished from its legal consequences. Questions of fact are decided by the jury, questions of law by the court or judge.
5. Philosophy: a proposition that may be either true or false, as contrasted with an evaluative statement.

If we look, we can easily see the subjectivity in each of these definitions. We end up back in Philosophy 101. The first: Known to have happened or existed—by whom? What is knowing? How is it that we know? Is general knowledge accepted? If so, then there are many formerly accepted facts, like the curative value of bloodletting or leeches, which have fallen by the wayside.

Or the second, "a truth, verifiable from experience or observation." We all know that experiential truth is obviously subjective. "I think it is too warm in here," says mom; "Are you kidding, it's freezing!" replies dad, to quote an actual example heard frequently in my parents' home. Observation requires an observer. Observers view things from their own subjective perspective.

The third, "a piece of information." Information does not imply truth. We are overloaded with information, much of it conflicting, sometimes diametrically opposed. This is the case in nutrition where many contrasting views exist. We can search the Web and find copious evidence for and against soy as a health food. There is as much or more information indicating that cholesterol is good for health than that it is bad. To me, the more interesting "fact" is which information reaches us and who benefits from it.

The fourth, the legal definition of fact, demonstrates that fact is subject to interpretation. The jury decides the facts. The facts did not rain down unalterably from heaven.

The fifth, the philosophical understanding, is the most honest. A fact is a proposition. It is a premise. And as we learned in Chapter Three, whoever defines the premises wins the argument.

Truth and facts are subjective. They are premises. Premises can have real consequences for individuals and for communities. If, in 1970, an all-white southern jury decided that it was a "fact" that James Black, a promising and gifted student, killed Nellie White then James faced life imprisonment or even death row. In recent years, many murder convictions, especially in racially charged cases, have been overturned because of DNA evidence coming to light that exonerated the prisoner. Innocent inmates who have spent long years in jail have been set free.

If we believe, because powerful corporations tell us it is "fact," that a global economy is a good economy, and that we should buy pre-packaged American culture, then our local economy will most likely suffer. Cheap goods produced in China with degrading environmental standards will appear to cost less than similar goods made down the road. If we are not slim, white, and blue-eyed we might begin to believe we are unattractive, as these are the prominent models of beauty in the media. If we do not live in a mansion like those seen on television, we might begin to believe we are poor.

Why am I writing all this? I know it seems as if I have digressed from my loving premises, but be patient for a moment. Spiritually, there has always been another understanding of the truth. This is the truth of inner knowing. It is the truth of the certainty in our heart. When we listen within we can be true to our inner voice and vision, choosing a life that expresses our divinity, our inner calling, and the infinite spirit that moves through our stream of life. This real truth cannot be verified by a system such as contemporary science that is less than itself, less than Wholeness. An isolated part cannot demonstrate the whole but can allude to it. Spiritual truth is an internal reality that can be cultivated in the fertile soil of the heart. And spiritual truth tells us to love our neighbor as our self, because that neighbor is our self.

But is a corporation our neighbor? Who do corporations love, and to whom do they listen? "Corporation" is an interesting term. Corporal means "of the body." Corporate is having a body. Corporations do not have bodies, although there are legal entities known as "corporate bodies." The word "incorporate" means to make physical, but corporations are not corporeal. They are legal fictions that grant the rights and ideally the responsibilities of living beings to fictional entities. This is what is meant by the term "corporate personhood."

There are "truths" that widen the gulf between our physical life and spiritual nature, and truths that bring us into a greater wholeness. For many years, my thoughts about the corporate giant Monsanto have been an outstanding teacher in the power of love versus fear. If we view corporations as evil, their evil aspects present themselves to our awareness. Then we can be at war with them and valiantly fight them—fight them in our neighborhoods as they pollute, fight them as they lobby for more control of natural resources, fight them for water. Fight them as farmers whose crops are contaminated by wind-pollinated GMO corn or alfalfa, farmers who are then sued by the contaminators for patent violation. Fight them for the gene pool of seeds and even the human genome.

This has been one of the most challenging areas for me personally. Should I love Monsanto? I can love rats, salmonella, and fleas, but Monsanto? It is not a living being. It is not an inanimate object like a rock or a crystal. It is not a force of nature like the wind or a natural phenomenon like a tsunami. In his brilliant satirical novels, Jasper Fforde creates the ultimate mega-corporation that he aptly names "Goliath." Fforde's Goliath is ruthless, self-serving, and diabolical. In my worst moments, that is certainly how I see Monsanto.

Because I observe myself I know that focusing negatively on corporations or on pharmaceutical companies hurts me. Corporations become another mirror of the self/other trap. In a dualistic system they are the "bad" guys, the ones who must change. But what if this is not the best way for me to look at the situation? What if focusing upon "bad" behavior somehow perpetuates it? Amplifies it? What if a belief that bad corporations do bad things creates an opportunity to get confirmatory evidence and impedes the flow of energy toward desired change? I feel stress, anxiety, and powerlessness when I focus on corporate misdeeds. When I think about these aspects of corporations, I exhibit little nervous tics like picking at my cuticles. My focus amplifies the qualities of these organizations that I definitely do not prefer. I attract more worrisome information, finding news reports to substantiate my fears. My fear feeds the fearfulness and feelings of powerlessness. It is just as I have been discussing throughout this book.

You get the picture. Still I believe, as did Anne Frank, that people are inherently good. We may think corporations are large, soulless, profit-driven behemoths, but they are made up of people—people with beliefs, aspirations, and desires like investors, shareholders, boards of directors, and workers. Corporations have cultures, and like any culture, they can shift. I choose not to hate microbes, and I would prefer not to hate big companies either. Hate, in any form, always diminishes. Hate is poisonous to the hater but has little or no effect on the hated. But I do not have to love them. I do not have to like what they do. The problem, if there is one, is in my giving my persistent attention to the unwanted. Judging and blaming become my problem because they keep me focused upon unhappiness. They keep me feeling discouraged and disempowered.

I struggled with this aspect of the Law of Attraction for a long time. Is it not valiant to fight oppression? This thorny issue comes out of the concept that Abraham-Hicks terms "contrast." Contrast is provided by situations that create desire for a new, improved situation. Contrast, says Abraham, "puts the eternalness in eternity." Contrast, that which is not wanted, actually helps to define what we do want. We benefit from noticing the things we do not like. So notice the things you do not want, such as power plays and manipulations, and then move on to your heart. There is no need to continue to focus on the problem or its cause. A solution is born as soon as we notice that improvement is desired.

When people are rude to you, you want respect. When you are rude to someone else, you want to be respectful. We only delay the desired change by staying focused on the problem. To shift, we must focus on solutions and be receptive to them. Answers and new perspectives come when we allow them in, from a new mindset. Let the heart's wisdom guide your actions. Focusing upon what gives us joy, where we find contentment, where we find peace and harmony sets the stage for resolutions, rebalancing, and epiphanies.

Corporations now purport to be ecological. Environmentalists refer to this as "green washing." They maintain that corporations are employing public relations ploys while continuing business as usual. I prefer to think that a corporation focusing upon its ecological image is a small but positive step. It indicates an acknowledgement that harmony with the Earth matters, and that this message is infiltrating their corporate culture. Whether corporations can actually step up to the challenge of being truly green is questionable, and also not my concern. Nature shows us that eventually those things that are far out of balance do not survive. Rapacious corporate cultures are not viable in the long term. There is no need to focus upon their misdeeds or to feel disempowered. Our goal is to make our personal choices from our hearts, understanding that we are empowered to create visionary worlds. Our day-to-day choices do make an enormous difference.

For example, if most people begin eating local, seasonal, and organic food, there will be far fewer pesticides sold. If most people and farmers choose diversity-enhancing heritage breeds of livestock, or heritage seeds, there will be fewer genetically modified organisms. Building local communities, supporting local artisans, caring for the biodiversity of your region all support a different economy. Think about what you value. After basic needs like food, clothing, and shelter are met, it is intangibles like friendship, fun, relationship, and community that people really care about. Do you want a homogenous planet with one dominant culture or do you appreciate the diversity of our world?

Shopping at the local farmers' market or buying direct from a farm share, you get the pleasure of developing a relationship with people who are raising your food. You also support a different economy, one where the people who raise the food actually know the people who eat it. Generally, there would be more personal responsibility in such a system. If I buy milk from farmer Lisa and she sees my kids thriving, then she will take pride in her product. She will also do everything in her power to ensure that the milk is as healthy and wholesome as possible, because she is a real person directly dealing with other real people. There would be less need for legislation in a closed loop such as this. People answer to their own hearts, and do their best. This type of exchange also keeps a lot more money in the local community. It can provide jobs and dollars for people you know, rather than faceless, nameless "shareholders."

My friend, the psychiatrist I mentioned previously, died of cancer before her fiftieth birthday. Her conflicted feelings about participating in the advisory panels was just one of many longstanding problems that gnawed at her. To honor her, to honor myself, I will choose a different path. I will not continue to live with painful contradictions swept under the rugs of my life.

So what is the answer to all this? One does not have to like everything in physical reality to connect with the stream of universal love.

Simply turn away from focus on that which feels disturbing. This is not the same as putting my head in the sand. It is possible to notice what I do not want and then turn my focus to things I prefer. I can build a new world, a new society from what feels good.

I start with noting my preferences. I prefer the feeling of well-being. I prefer feeling whole-hearted and not guilty about my choices. I prefer community. I prefer thriving local economies. I prefer pristine environments. I prefer spending time in nature, hearing the dawn chorus of bird song and marveling at the chevron flight of geese. I prefer clean air, clean water, and rich healthy soil. I prefer diverse ecosystems. I prefer seeing a world where more people are living life fully and consciously as the spiritual beings they are. I prefer finding meaning and pleasure in my work. I prefer caring for my neighbor as myself.

Noting our preferences helps us define action. What to do? Point the arrow of your internal compass toward what you want. Suspend trying to "figure it out" and move to the primacy of the intelligence of the heart. The search for truth is a chimera. Most "truth" is illusory, a construct of the mind. It is a construct of politics and vested interests that do not necessarily share my values. Truth, as presented to us, is not of the heart.

In *As You Like It*, Shakespeare wrote these famous lines: "All the world's a stage, / And all the men and women merely players: / They have their exits and their entrances; / And one man in his time plays many parts, ..." Corporations today can be seen as playing the role of villain. In doing so, they help us to see that our communities and ecosystems matter deeply, and that the best things in life aren't things. Corporations help people to notice one another, to see the value in societies and nature.

I predict that society will continue to change and improve. We already see evidence of that change. We can learn to gently enhance and support nature by working with natural processes. We are already developing many technologies that are in harmony with nature and our planet. We can live in a whole-hearted manner. We can apply the power of our thoughts and minds in union with our hearts. We can be motivated by love, not fear. We can step out of the whole game of right and wrong and live more and more in the unity of our true nature. Jalal al-din Rumi, the thirteenth-century Sufi poet and mystic, said: "There is a field, beyond ideas of right doing and wrong doing. I'll meet you there."

That field is the field of heart truth. It is the field of knowing who we really are. It is the field where we are one, like the vast networks of mycorrhizae. It is the minerals that form our bones and flesh today, recycled remnants of dying, exploding stars from eons past. Be aware. Look around at what you love, and let your love guide you.

Tools for Transformation

1. Continuing with breathing exercises, we notice that we can breathe love and well-being anywhere to anyone at any time. This is a very expansive exercise, full of possibilities. We can be beacons of love and well-being and can radiate this love energy anywhere. We can send it to corporate boardrooms, crippled nuclear reactors, marine life, and coastal communities struggling with massive oil spills or the after-effects of tsunamis. In doing so, we are sending love to ourselves.

   How? First, consciously step out of any feelings of alarm, and center in the peace of your heart. Breathe in, breathe out. Include a word in your breathing if that helps you toward well-being. Peace, ease, freedom, love are all nice words, but choose something that soothes you. Breathe in peace, out peace, in freedom, out freedom. There is a bigger picture you are tuning to, one beyond dualism. Let go of thoughts. Acknowledge them when they arise, but let them go. See them as little bubbles floating away or wispy clouds dispersed by a gentle wind. If needed, just soothe yourself. When you have an overall feeling of ease, joy, comfort, and fullness you might breathe in to your heart, and with your out-breath allow your love to flow to where it is needed. Then breathe in through that area and out through your own heart.

2. Here's a practical example. Perhaps you are concerned about the ongoing nuclear contamination at the Fukushima reactors in Japan. Worrying feels terrible, so you know it is not a good track for you. Center instead in your heart. Take some time to feel the wholeness. There is no need to hurry. Let your breath be easy. Breathe in well-being, out well-being. When you feel a sense of knowing of something bigger than your individual life right now, when you feel love, wholeness, and comfort, breathe this in to your heart. Then staying with the same sense of knowing, breathe well-being, the understanding of a greater whole, to Fukushima. Breathe love to the people of Japan, the earth, the ocean, and the radioactive elements themselves. Breathe love in through them then back out again through your own heart.

This is a powerful technique for healing. In doing this, you are focusing a dynamic beam of love, wholeness, and well-being that benefits all.

—CHAPTER THIRTEEN—

The Spirits of Things

MANY SOCIETIES AND RELIGIONS ACKNOWLEDGE that other living beings such as trees, flowers, and insects have spirits. This same understanding applies to natural elements like wind, rain, clouds, mountains, rivers, and stones. Qualities such as compassion and love are associated with various deities. The goddess Quan Yin of traditional Chinese culture is associated with compassion and holds a position similar to that of the Virgin Mary in Catholicism. In Greek mythology Aphrodite was associated with physical beauty, and in contemporary society we still metaphorically associate Cupid's arrows with love. New Age devotees ascribe physical, emotional, and esoteric properties to various crystals and minerals. In societies where these spirits are acknowledged, communication with them is endorsed and encouraged. In the currently dominant society, the spirits of things are recognized only in a metaphorical or imaginary sense. They are mentioned in poetry, literature, mythology, and folklore. "Zeus wielded a thunderbolt." "The wind whispered my name."

The idealized understanding (and subsequent personalization) of any higher life form or natural element is commonly referred to as a *deva*. The term *deva* derives from the Sanskrit root *diw*, which means "shining, luminous, or radiant." The terms Deity, Divine, and Divinity, as well as the term for God in many languages (such as Dios in Spanish and Dieu in French) all derive from this Sanskrit root. Even the God-name Zeus derives from this Sanskrit term for divinity. The term for a Goddess is Devi. The modern-day word "diva," applied to talented female performers in music and the arts, is derived from this same root.

In Hinduism, devas are divine non-physical angelic-type beings who represent the natural and moral forces present in the physical world. There are major and minor devas. But just like in Western religions, there is only one Supreme Being or God. Devas can be seen as either servants of one great Divinity or aspects of it. This is similar to the manner in which humans and human life express aspects of the Divine.

"Elementals" is another term used to describe certain aspects of the spirit of things. Elementals are particular types of nature spirits common in folklore. Elementals take many forms, categorized by the four alchemical elements: air, earth, fire, and water. All elementals can be willful or playful, helpful or destructive. In folklore, air elementals are sylphs who draw cloud pictures and direct winds and storms. Water elementals are undines. They calm the waters and sing to sailors but also stir the waters at their whim. Fire elementals are salamanders. Firefighters will tell you how fire seems to have a mind of its own. Earth elementals are gnomes. They can be grumpy or friendly, garden gnomes who help growing things, troll-like grouches, or wise and friendly teachers.

While the term "deva" originated in the Hindu world, the contemporary understanding of it has expanded beyond Hindu characterization. Now people of diverse traditions speak of devas, elementals, and nature spirits. One way to understand the devic realm is as a reservoir of wisdom that holds the sacred template for each type of being. Devas are overarching spirits or archetypes that can appear physical and represent the natural world to us. Many people, especially children, have reported interactions (usually playful) with devas, animal spirits, totems, and elementals. Communication with devas is possible, especially during expanded and altered states of consciousness. There is a deva of roses and a deva of oceans. Even forces of nature like wind and rain have an intelligence and consciousness with which we can communicate.

It is interesting to note that a maternal Goddess figure has appeared to people throughout recorded history, offering comfort and nurturance and sometimes physical and emotional healing. The early Catholic Church was very interested in sites where she frequently appeared. The most potent and reliable of these became sites associated with Mary, and cathedrals were built upon them. The site of the Virgin of Guadalupe in Mexico was one that was sacred to the Toltec people.

In his writings, author Malidoma Somé describes, from an insider's perspective, the many ways that his people, the Dagara of Western Africa, traditionally communicate with spirits of nature. Native Americans also communicate with elements of nature. Animal spirits become totems for individuals and clans. Forces of nature are understood to be conscious entities with which communication is possible. Maria Sabina was a Native medicine woman in Mexico who healed with the help of the spirits she encountered in sacred mushrooms. There were consistent beings she saw again and again in her journeys.

My first conscious interaction with nature spirits or devas occurred when I was five or six years old. A weeping willow tree grew on a neighbor's property near our home. I loved this willow. Her graceful branches swept the earth and I could hide beneath them, resting against the sturdy trunk. Sheltered there, I had my own special secret spot but could still hear my mom if she called for me. Although I got along well with neighborhood kids, I never told them about my hideaway because I liked to be alone with the willow. I knew the willow loved me and that we were friends.

One day other children wanted to cut some of the willow's slender branches and make switches from them to swat at each other. I did not like this and encouraged them to play other games. I felt pain at the thought of them cutting her branches; I saw her bleeding sap from her injury and it felt quite uncomfortable to me. Plus, I knew she did not want to be part of a taunting game. I was able to persuade the other kids that this was not a good idea, downplaying the fun they expected and explaining that "getting hit with switches hurts a lot, and your parents will be really mad if you come home bleeding." They moved on and I stayed with my willow, pretending I had to go home soon.

Now surely this all could have been my projection, but at five years of age I felt the extraordinary relationship clearly, in a manner distinct from the way I related to other trees. The willow had a unique personality and was definitely a she. She felt reliable, dependable, and calm. After that day, the willow would talk to me when I was sheltered under her bower. I do not recall if I perceived words, but I do remember that her communication could be very funny and downright silly. This was a very stressful time for my family, and she would comfort me when I was sad or upset. There was a quality of light under the willow that I came to rely upon, and this light was my first conscious doorway into the Green World.

What was happening here? Can a willow tree really speak? At five years old I didn't know that most people did not hear trees, so I was free to have my experience. I had many friends growing up, both physical and non-physical. They all seemed normal to me. My parents called the non-physical ones that they could not see "imaginary friends." To their credit, they never discouraged my interactions with these friends. I wasn't sure what "imaginary" meant, so I made up my own definition that had more to do with the kind of people they were. I could clearly perceive them, but I could tell that there was a difference between the friends my parents described as imaginary and the other children I knew from the neighborhood. My imaginary friends were very diverse and most did not look like people. Some looked like vegetables with faces, some looked like pictures in fairy tale books, and others looked like wavy lines.

Amazing doors open when we are aware that it is possible to communicate directly with the spirits of things. Flower and vibrational essences are one example of healing tools born of an expanded understanding of interrelatedness. Essences are vibrational impressions of a flower, leaf, gem, or other entity, stabilized in water and pre-served with grape alcohol or another neutral medium. Essences have been used extensively in healing by various cultures as a form of spirit medicine. Essences were possibly important tools in ancient human societies such as those of Egypt and Sumeria, as well as in fabled so-cieties like Atlantis and Lemuria of which there is no certain physical record.

More recently, Dr. Edward Bach reintroduced essences to the heal-ing repertory. Bach was a successful London homeopath in the early twentieth century. Due to a crisis of faith in his work, he came to believe that even homeopathy did not address the spiritual roots of illness. Bach believed that illness was caused by "a contradiction be-tween the purposes of the soul and the personality's point of view." He left his practice to become a wanderer in the countryside, com-muning intuitively with trees and plants and often sleeping outdoors. During this period, he gave away his services for free to those who requested them. Through communication with the natural world, he evolved the original thirty-eight Bach flower essences. These essences are made from typical plants of the British countryside in the early twentieth century.

Since that time many other essences have been made from native plants of other areas. The world of essences has expanded beyond flow-ers as well. There are falling leaf essences, gem elixirs, planetary and starlight essences, environmental and seasonal essences, animal essenc-es, and more. Any aspect of nature can teach us about balance and har-mony as we communicate with it and acknowledge its consciousness.

Vibrational tools are not necessary for healing, but for many peo-ple they are beneficial. They can help us to focus positively, giving attention to desired outcomes of well-being and greater harmony in various areas of our life. By focusing on what we intend, we gently release our resistance to and disbelief in the desired outcome. We inform our subconscious of our new directional heading.

Essences are useful tools for restoring balance on mental, emotional, and spiritual levels. They are created intuitively, with the active cooperation and participation of the elements of the natural world. They connect the spirit of the plants, flowers, trees, animals, stars, gems, etc., with the individual or group who is experiencing imbalance or misunderstanding. How does this happen? These other forms of consciousness do not have the level of resistance that we, as complex thinking creative beings, can aggregate. They can assist us because they are already in harmony. They can help us see our natural state of relaxation and well-being. It is often easier to see our limiting beliefs while working with essences. I find them especially helpful in revealing ingrained patterns, learned perhaps from family or society, that no longer serve growth or well-being. They are powerful but benign tools assisting the restoration of communication between the higher self/soul and the personality.

Essences are gentle. Unlike medications and especially pharmaceuticals, there is no possibility of causing symptoms associated with disharmony. They do not push or force change but rather invite it in. Essences work in harmony with a greater soul-plan of the being who uses them. If an essence used is not necessary at a specific time, nothing happens. If one is using combination essences, only those appropriate for the individual at the time they are taken will be active.

While essences are subtle, this does not mean they are weak or ineffective. On the contrary, I have found essences to be among the most powerful tools of awakening and allowing that I have utilized. The effects are more noticeable as we quiet down and are able to connect with the inner self. Tools such as journaling and meditation help us observe and amplify the benefits of essences. Physical and emotional changes may ensue, as patterns of disharmony dissolve and the self becomes more knowing of its essential nature. Sometimes essences can help us connect with an understanding of the roots of disharmony that led to a physical ailment or imbalance. As we are able to release this misunderstanding we can gradually observe beneficial effects in physical health.

In my work, I have found essences particularly useful for highly sensitive people who are unable to take other types of remedies. For example, I had one patient, a woman I'll call Amanda, who was in her early thirties when she first consulted with me. Amanda suffered from anxiety, severe shyness, and agoraphobia. While she was not a danger to herself or others (situations we are taught to evaluate in medical training), she certainly was lonely and depressed. She had sought help from numerous physicians and natural healers but could not tolerate pharmaceuticals, herbs, or homeopathic remedies. She was helped by psychotherapy but was not working with it when we had our visit because of financial difficulties. Pharmaceutical drugs made her jittery, nauseated, headachy, and spaced out. She had dog-gedly tried more than thirty medications, in many classes of drugs, but all gave overwhelming side effects. Even herbs and individual nutri-ents caused her an unacceptable level of discomfort.

Amanda heard of me through a friend and was ready for a different approach. She believed her physical and emotional problems could be overcome and had some sense that there was a deeper meaning to what she was experiencing. For example, she wanted self-acceptance but realized that she was usually self-critical. She also knew she wanted to worry less. She catastrophized even minor events, and she equated possibility, however remote, with probability.

Over a period of months Amanda's treatment program consisted of essences, meditation, breathing exercises, and slight changes in her diet. All of these felt good to her. Because of her finances, we met infrequently. Improvements were noticeable, however, even af-ter our first visit. Amanda gradually became calmer, catastrophizing less and exhibiting a sweet sense of humor when she did veer again into old familiar territory. She utilized the essences as a vehicle for focusing upon the positive changes she was ready to make. I adjusted her essences each visit depending upon what was up for her. Often a shift of essences was the only thing we did during a visit. Working gently in this manner was profound for Amanda. With the assistance of the essences, combined with self-examination tools, she found herself able to unravel old dysfunctional patterns and begin healthy new ones. Three years and many essences later, Amanda is no longer agoraphobic and only mildly anxious at times. She is working in a small, low-key office with co-workers she likes. Her finances have improved a great deal since she now can comfortably leave her home and go to work. She was recently married and seems very happy.

I am well aware that discussion of the spirits within things moves us well out of the realm of conventional science. Materialist scientists might dismiss the benefits of flower essences as "just" a placebo effect. But that still begs the question of how to explain placebo effect? Placebos, in fact, are powerful medicines. Researchers refer to their effects as the "placebo problem." They are factored into drug trials because twenty-five to seventy percent of individuals will improve using placebo alone. Dr. Herbert Benson of Harvard University believes this may be as high as ninety percent in some situations.[1] This is twenty-five to seventy percent above the number that would improve anyway if there were no intervention of any sort.

Some research indicates that the bigger and more elaborate the placebo, the greater the likelihood of success. For example, sham operations have been done as part of studies on placebo effect. In one small but well-known study done at the Veterans' Administration Hospital in Houston in 1994, Dr. Bruce Moseley worked with a group of ten patients with arthritic knee pain. The patients consented to be part of a study, and all knew they would have either a real or a sham operative procedure. In fact, only two had the full arthroscopic knee surgery, three had a washing of the inside of the knee joint (one part of arthroscopic surgery), and five merely had three flesh cuts around the knee to simulate the appearance of an operation, but no actual surgery of any sort was performed. All ten reported significant improvement in their pain after the "operation." Even six months later, all the patients were satisfied with the outcomes of their "surgeries." The study was repeated with a larger group, 180 patients, and the results, published in 2002 in the distinguished journal *The New England Journal of Medicine,* found no difference in outcomes for patients who had real arthroscopic surgery versus placebo.[2] In the United States, placebo pills used to be available for prescription but were eventually deemed unethical except for clinical trials and are no longer available. So even "hard science" acknowledges that something is happening with placebos, causing a "placebo problem" that is yet another elephant in the living room leading us to the tricky role of mind and consciousness.

From the new premise that we are spiritual beings, sparks of divinity, creators, it is easy to see that the magic in the placebo is us. The power of placebo is the power of belief, the power of focus. The more we believe, the better the outcome. That may well be the power of many drugs and even vitamins. The earliest trials of SSRI antidepressants like Fluoxetine (well known as the brand Prozac®) and Sertraline (well known as the brand Zoloft®) were disappointing due to the meager benefits demonstrated by the drugs. But as more prescriptions were written and more doctors believed in them, they, like Tinker Bell, grew magically stronger. Later trials of the same drugs, which by then were popular and widely accepted, showed much more robust benefits.

Spirit will reflect to us the sum of our beliefs. One way of thinking about pharmaceuticals and drug manufacturers is seeing them as an evil empire. They may be thought of as a necessary evil, yet one rife with excesses that require constant vigilance. Within this viewpoint, drug manufacturers are self-serving. They promote false health and bilk us of our money. In this view, too often drugs are harmful things that cause unnatural disasters like two-headed frogs. We see

this stream of thought reflected to us in the Bhopal disaster, in tragedies like Thalidomide, in actual two-headed frogs and other alarming
aberrations found increasingly in the effluent streams from chemical
and pharmaceutical plants. One can find lots of gruesome evidence
to support this case. Since we attract what we focus upon, it is not
surprising that people who focus upon the evils of chemicals and
pharmaceuticals easily attract evidence to support their beliefs.

Another perspective sees pharmaceuticals as modern saviors and
as solid blue-chip investments. In this camp the wonders of modern
miracle drugs are touted in glowing glossy advertisements. My parents, bless them, are of this perspective. They believe in doctors and
prescription drugs. They heavily utilize the whole system. My dad[3]
is on about twenty medications and my mom uses eight. Neither is
in good health, though they are satisfied with their medical care. My
mom quipped recently that she and dad are spending their old age
together going to medical appointments and hospitals.

I straddle the fence. I notice that modern medicine is extolled
even as it produces lackluster benefits. An equal number of people
die from miracle cures and simple medications as are cured by them.
Non-steroidal anti-inflammatory drugs have killed more people than
the many who have died from AIDS. Many over-the-counter medications like acetaminophen (a pain reliever) and phenylpropanolamine
(a common cough suppressant) are known to cause serious and even
fatal complications. It is widely acknowledged that at least one quarter million people die in the United States every year from iatrogenic
(medically caused) diseases, and much of this is from pharmaceuticals.[4] This makes iatrogenic illness the third leading cause of death in
the U.S. after cardiovascular disease and cancer. This is more than five
times as many people as are killed in automobile accidents![5] Some
people, esteemed physicians included, estimate that when all medically related deaths are counted, modern medicine is the number-one
leading cause of mortality.[6]

But I also see that there are many choices in the medical world that do alleviate suffering. My partner Star had pneumonia a few years ago and took a course of antibiotics that swiftly cleared the infection. Before that she was so short of breath that she felt winded just walking a flight of stairs. This caused me to think of all those long convalescing illnesses described in seventeenth-century literature. Some ailments that once took months to resolve can be swiftly cured today.

I was inspired to build a career in medicine by my desire to be of service to others. I gravitated toward natural healing since I did not like the idea of running to doctors or taking a pill for every ill. As I came to understand more about the role of consciousness, I thought about it in relationship to medicines. Consider that pharmaceuticals are not outside the spirit of things. Everything, even human creations, has some sort of spirit or vibration. It is interesting to consider how we might energetically communicate with medicines. If there is no place where I end and you begin, then our I–thou relationship extends not only to the groovy natural things like plants, waterfalls, and crystals but also to asphalt, pharmaceuticals, and the works of our hands. If we want medications with a soul, we have to allow them a soul. Consider dialogue with them too.

We are the miracles, not the drugs. To use a Biblical metaphor, today's drugs are like a Golden Calf, made by us and misguidedly worshiped as divine. I propose a new model. Pharmaceuticals are tools. They are our own creation. That does not make them unworthy. We are divine creators in our own right. In the past few centuries, medicines have often been created from our fear, made without conscious connection to our love or to our hearts. Pharmaceuticals were developed as soldiers in the war against disease. Their roots were disconnected from love, so it is not surprising that the end result, medications deeply out of balance with the planet, reflect the beginnings. But what if drug companies were benevolent? What if they were run and staffed by people who had the well-being of the whole in their hearts and minds? If you believe this is possible, then you are more likely to experience it in your lifetime.

If we embody love in the creation of medicines, what can we make? One example is spagyric medicines—natural medicines, both herbal and homeopathic, made from an alchemical process developed by a mystic and physician, Paracelsus, in the sixteenth century. Paracelsus was a prominent European physician in his era. He lived and worked just a hundred years prior to the seventeenth-century separation of science and spirit. In the sixteenth century one could still be both a physician and a healer. Respected physicians could be alchemists.

Popular culture portrays alchemy as the quixotic quest to transform base metals into gold. But the inner teachings of alchemy are about the transformation of the soul. The path of transforming ordinary souls of ordinary people into the golden souls of enlightened masters is the real journey of the alchemist. Alchemy is a methodology for assisting everyday people in strengthening the conscious connection of their inner being with their physical existence. Alchemy maintains that a Divine Golden soul resides in each of us. Alchemically, we learn to express our real natures more and more. So, in making spagyric medicines, all aspects of a substance are used so that the medicine operates on all levels: physical, emotional, and spiritual. There are now several lines of spagyric homeopathic medicines and herbal compounds available commercially.

Love in medicine is not a new concept, nor is love in food. Most of us believe that the meal that grandma lovingly prepares for her family is special. Some people even say it is made with "vitamin L." I imagine that most medicines made with "vitamin L" are natural, created by mimicry and enhancement of nature. A popular adage of the 1960s was: "We are building the new society in the vacant lots of the old." The buildings going up in the vacant lots of medicine are found in the arena of nature-derived medicine and remedies. An enormous amount has already been built in this expanding market. Through listening to the voice of nature in her various forms we can conceive more tools to strengthen and enhance life. Nature will then happily show us how to include "vitamin L" in our curative compounds.

Tools for Transformation:
Observing the Heart-Fields of Others

1. The ability to watch energetically is available to anyone who dedicates herself to the task. By gently and non-judgmentally watching the heart-fields of others, we can notice the clarity of the communication between the divine self and the physical human. We can position ourselves in the place of clarity of communication and simply rest there, offering our awareness of wholeness and well-being. By merely observing compassionately, we help others to strengthen their connections to their inner being.

   Begin by centering in your own heart with your breath. When you have a sense of serenity and connection with your heart, gently shift your gaze to the heart-field of the person you are observing. This may be at their breast-bone but can extend several feet from the body as well. Let your gaze be loose, your mind easy. Hold an intention of good for the person you are observing. You are not looking for problems and do not need a laser-like focus. Allow impressions to come in whatever way they do. Stay in your own feelings of calm and serenity. Find and know the place where the other person is fine just as they are. Embody that wholeness and rest there.

2. Practice letting go of analyzing your observations. Impressions come exponentially faster than the interpretive brain can process. Merely notice what it is that you notice, staying in the flow of impressions, as if you are flowing effortlessly in a moving current.

3. When beginning to learn this technique, it is most helpful to look at the hearts of babies and very small children. Their hearts are pure. They are close to the light from which we all were born. When you look, it is easy to see the well-being in them. Newborn babies practically glow. This aura is all around them but is especially apparent at the heart. The heart-field of infants can be very wide, extending many feet from their bodies. Remember that observation does not have to be visual. We all perceive in our own ways. Your way of observing may be a peaceful or exultant feeling, or you may have a sense of knowing, or be aware of some sort of sound. Let yourself be free as you explore, holding the finest and purist of intentions for those you observe, including when you observe yourself. When we observe the light in others, our own light shines more clearly.

—CHAPTER FOURTEEN—

The Deva of Fleas

There are two ways to live: you can live as if nothing is a
miracle; you can live as if everything is a miracle.

—ALBERT EINSTEIN

IN THE SUMMER OF 2009, during a meditation journey, the Deva of
Fleas visited me. My eyes were closed when she arrived, an immense flea giantess, much larger than me. She sat serenely in my internal field of view, filling the screen of my inner images and simply
waited. I knew why she was there. The proverbial chickens had come
home to roost. Her presence was divinely gentle. The only demand
she made was in the persistence of her patient waiting. I could not
escape. She would stay until I was ready.

This loving Devic visitation occurred several months after my
transformational experience with the ants. I suppose I knew some
sort of reckoning was coming, but I had no idea how to resolve my
contradictions. I was ready for some help. For many years in various
ways, I had felt pestered by fleas. While I did not hate fleas, I could not
be said to love them either. I did love them in the abstract, as essence,
as I love all consciousness, all life. But I was a flea killer.

I acknowledged readily to the Deva that I was not killing fleas
for my nourishment or so that I might live. I was not slaughtering
them as a participant in the sacred mystery of the circle of life
nourishing life. No, I was killing them out of fear and annoyance,
fears of inconvenience, irritating bites, and itching. Fear, ultimately,
that I could not walk my talk. I was ashamed of murdering fleas and
felt bad each time I did it. A rash of justifications inundated in my
mind, but none of these resonated with my heart. It is amusing how
consciousness eventually brings us back to our little inconsistencies

on the "purify our hearts to serve Thee in truth" side of the equation.

At that time in 2009, my current experience with fleas was one of relative peace. To use the war metaphor, it resembled a low-level cease-fire with occasional outbreaks of skirmishing. There was certainly not true harmony. As she sat and waited, I had to acknowledge this as well. I still felt upset by fleas. I disliked them. I did not want them around. I did not feel resolved about my thoughts and emotions about fleas. Thoughts of "why do they have to exist at all" commingled with "all beings have a place and purpose." Where I sat on the fence was a barometer of my moment-to-moment level of connectedness with the greater whole.

My partner Star would occasionally laugh at me. The more I focused upon fleas, the more I noticed fleas in our home. Star never had flea-bites. The dog and cat seemed largely untroubled as well, though it was easy for me to spot the odd flea crawling on my sandy-colored pooch. Even at a distance, I seemed to have a radar lock fixated upon sighting flea movements on our dog Lily. In our little family, this issue was mine alone, though Lily occasionally obliged with a mini-infestation. By then we "managed" fleas mostly by the "non-toxic" (to us) method of frequent flea combing combined with aggressive vacuuming. While this introduced no pesticides into our home, it meant I was still personally and frequently assassinating fleas by combing them out of Lily's fur, then drowning them in little soapy dishes of water. Our cat Jerry, on the other hand, would have none of this. I could not even get one swipe of the flea comb down her soft grey back without her hissing in protest and nipping my hand reprovingly.

My flea odyssey began in my late teens, during my second year of college. I lived in an off-campus house with two other students, three big dogs, and very little vacuuming. The emotional context for this period of my life was a turbulence that expressed itself in many ways. I was in my first romantic relationship, of which my parents knew nothing, for I knew they would sharply disapprove of my choice.

Even I grew unsure of my choice, for my own reasons, but did not know how to break up, because I was mortified at the thought of hurting my kind boyfriend's feelings.

I felt conflicted during that time for various other reasons as well. I actually did not want to be in college at all that year. I really had desperately wanted a gap year but felt unable to stand up to my parents' insistence that I plod on. They were adamantly opposed to my plan of a year of work and travel, vowing they would not continue to pay for my education if I took any time off. I felt railroaded and powerless.

This period of my life was marked by overall feelings of striving, without any sense of faith in my capacity to achieve. I knew I was smart and academically gifted, but this didn't seem to add up to any feelings of self-confidence outside the classroom.

I knew I did not want to end up with a mediocre or even average life. I felt a flame inside of me, and yet I had a lot of growing up and differentiating from my parents to do. I felt I had some important calling, but I had no sense of how to get there from my position of somewhat low self-esteem.

Our little cottage developed a major "flea problem" and I was the main one being bitten. At one point I had hundreds of bites covering my ankles and legs that eventually converged into one enormous welt. I sported many smaller inflamed patches on my torso and arms. I grew "allergic" to flea bites, and my scratching them would quickly elicit further swelling and oozing. I got a flea collar for my dog but did not feel comfortable with it. I was already suspicious of the chemical model of "pest control," and anyway, this was way too little, too late. Finally we "flea-bombed" our house twice in a two-week period, which certainly helped clear the manifestation of infestation, but my discomfort continued. I felt uneasy about the choice to use pesticides. Waiting outside in my car for the chemical mist to clear, I amplified my disquiet by recalling my childhood uneasiness about the DDT-laden "No Pest Strips" my parents hung in the kitchen and the backyard, and my knowledge that they were eventually banned as toxic. I even recalled my misgivings about the word "pests." I knew, for me, there was something really awry about the whole state of affairs, but this awareness just bolstered my general feelings of disempowerment. In those years I had no sense of how to listen to my emotions for guidance about a better-feeling way. In hindsight, I now see how much good came of that youthful, angst-ridden period of my life. In wishing for more, for a different way to see the whole, I was sowing the seeds of a future relationship with the natural world, and specifically with insects, based on cooperation and mutual respect. I was sowing the seeds of my own wholeness that would come to fruition as I grew in self-acceptance and self-awareness.

Though I deeply love animals, I was so traumatized by my flea experience that I did not get a pet again for twenty years. I still managed to magnetize occasional flea bites at other people's homes, even if they were unaware of fleas in their environment. Meanwhile, the fleas themselves just went about their business, living their lives. I hated them long after I felt uncomfortable about hating anything, because I felt plagued and powerless. Their presence felt invasive and unwelcome, but I did not encounter them often enough to focus upon shifting my way of looking at them. I certainly did not consider the possibility that the fleas were magnifying for me, at various points of my life, feelings and thoughts of powerlessness in many concurrent situations.

I adopted a puppy eleven years ago and was immediately confronted by the flea question. By then I was a holistic health physician. I ate organic food. I could not even have comfortably opened one of the flea collar packets, or touched a collar, let alone put one upon a dog I loved. In any case, flea collars were no longer popular, having been supplanted by oral and topical flea poisons now euphemistically referred to as medications. I loftily thought of myself as striving to have compassion for all living beings. To be honest, at that point I was not really including the fleas in my universal love, though the inconsistency occasionally tickled at the back of my mind.

Still, I let myself ignore my pesky contradictions while I focused on how to have a flea-free environment. Even while discounting the consciousness of fleas, I found no satisfactory solutions. For a brief time I tried those chemicals you place on the back of your pet once a month. True, they are effective in killing fleas, but I did not have ease about applying potent neurotoxins to animals that I love. Nor did I want to pet the dog while this stuff was soaking in during its monthly applications. The packages are very convincing about the importance of humans avoiding skin contact with the chemicals. I pondered the absurdity of accepting that it was okay for me to gob this stuff, once a month, on a small beloved animal, being sure to let it absorb fully down to their skin without washing them for days afterward, while knowing I immediately needed to thoroughly wash my hands if even a drop got on me. There is such a profound disconnect in this that I do not think I need to say more. I finally settled, uneasily, upon the once-a-month oral flea "medications." The package described them as a quaint form of flea "birth control." I saw the irony that these were not medications "for" the fleas—they were weapons of mass flea destruction, and flea forced-sterilization programs—but I felt my hands were tied. Sound familiar?

"Fleas are bad, aren't they?" I argued with myself. "They are *vermin*, like cockroaches, ticks, Lyme spirochetes, and rats." But I wasn't buying this, because I understood well by now that everything in my experience was about my relationship with my self, my inner self. Everything in my experience was my creation, because my focus and beliefs in some way brought it there.

While the Deva sat amiably with me, I finally admitted that fleas, too, are representative of some parts of my vibration. No longer my predominant vibration, true, but they portrayed some persistent and familiar themes. Frankly, I felt relief. I wanted to feel better, to feel aligned with myself. So I sat with the patient flea Deva and asked myself without recrimination: what do the fleas mirror to me? What does my attitude about them teach me about myself? I began with acknowledgment of my feelings about fleas—irritation, annoyance, and frustration. I recognized that these emotions were all too familiar.

The fleas reminded me of the ways I bite at myself. I do this more than I like to admit. Though much of my life is joyous, I nag and pressure myself to perform even at times when my heart is not in it. I second-guess myself too. Even when I've made a decision from a very centered place, and know it, I can later come back from a place of less alignment and pick my decision apart. That never felt comfortable, but it was a persistent pattern.

My physical reaction to flea bites reminded me of the ways I could inflame little worrisome things, blowing them out of proportion. I saw the ways I looked for problems and focused upon what might be wrong, just as I scrutinize my dog for any signs of flea movements. I maintained vigilance, and with it went an expectation that I would find irritating little things to annoy me.

As I considered the sacred role of these "pests," I began to feel a sense of amusement. What if fleas, rats, cockroaches, bedbugs, and other so-called vermin interface with us merely as messengers of the Divine? Persistently and doggedly calling us back on track.... I understood that like my Deva of Fleas, the vermin and the super-bugs are not going anywhere else until we look at ourselves and get into right relationship. Because they are our guests, they dwell in our experience at our vibrational invitation.

I shifted as I considered the meaning of my emotions about fleas. I slowly began to feel grateful to them for what I learn about myself. I appreciated their persistence in reminding me of my toleration of feelings of annoyance and self-doubt so prevalent that I barely noticed them anymore. There are times now, not always, that I actually love fleas. I love them with amusement, as I am learning to love "all my creations," with the understanding that any thing in my experience is my creation. The Deva affably sat with me through this entire journey. We spent over an hour together in my room on the first day, and she appeared frequently through the following month as I worked through my issues.

A further confirmation of my transformation came a few weeks later in a lucid dream. In it, I went to the great sanctuary of Rats. Their shrine was a resplendent temple-like tent palace, seemingly located in India, and filled with the finest carpets. The Rat King had invited me there as an honored guest. Outside this structure there were hundreds of rats, coming and going. I was aware of a mythic, epic quality throughout the experience. I entered slowly. Entering of my own volition, in trust, was a first test that I somehow passed. Inside, the tent was festooned with brightly hued pennants in a rainbow of colors. There were thousands of rats everywhere, scurrying along the floor, perched on rafters, and snuggled together on rich brocaded furnishings. There was great diversity among them: big rats, tiny rats, black, brown, speckled, and white ones, little pink-nosed lab rats, and huge urban brown rats. I was initially a little overwhelmed: and even in this dream state, I had a knee-jerk queasiness in the pit of my stomach. But I felt no sense of malice from the rats who were just going about their sacred business.

I did not push past my fears and trepidation. Instead, I calmed myself, breathing in and out through my heart. I recognized a feeling of amused warmth and curiosity emanating from the rats. I was an esteemed visitor—my presence had been respectfully requested and I had graciously responded with a matching respect and tentative trust. Apparently this was not a frequent occurrence, and the rats were pleased. Still, I traversed cautiously, both to avoid inadvertently injuring any of them by stepping upon them, and to maintain my equilibrium and not freak out as I moved deeper into their territory. This seemed to be a second test that I also passed, for just beyond the mid-point, I sensed an energetic shift in the temple that amplified my increasing feelings of calm. The sea of rats parted before each footfall. I strode slowly to the back of the tent, where the Rat King awaited. He was very large and solemn, a Deva as well, I am sure, though inexplicably not quite as large as my new friend, the Deva of Fleas. I smiled and extended my hand, and he extended his paw. The third and final test had been passed. A look of deep peace and understanding traversed the gap of our shared gaze, and then, like an electrical impulse across a synapse, some sort of energetic exchange occurred via our touch that stirred the core of my being. I felt I had peered into the loving eyes of Hanuman, the enlightened monkey deity of the Hindu pantheon, and found myself within them. No words were spoken. I then awoke fully, with a clear memory of the entire sequence. I felt enveloped by a love as immeasurable as any I have ever known—a love that once again mirrored the Golden World to me. Though it took place in a dream, this interaction was so profound that I still cannot tell this story or even re-read it without weeping.

Today my level of comfort with fleas varies. When I am most disconnected, I still worry about the fleas a bit, but then I breathe and relax, breathe and find ease. After thus soothing myself, I can glimpse a sweet laughing Deva out of the corner of my eye. Not surprisingly, there are not many actual physical fleas in my experience. I have not spotted any in months on my dog (though I do not scrutinize either), and neither dog nor cat is scratching herself unduly. Two years have passed without a flea bite.

When I am my most connected, I find fleas amusing. I feel deep gratitude to them, and especially to the Deva of Fleas, who sought me out and helped me in so many ways. I am now more patient with myself. When I am not in the mood for something, I do not just ignore my feelings of discomfort and power through; I take time to find my center. Either I go ahead and let myself joyously do something more appealing, despite my "should," or I find the delight in what I have agreed upon as my responsibility.

I do not look for problems. I do not try to discover ways that patients, friends, and relatives are not thriving because they are not conforming to the way I think things should be done. I focus on what feels better. This has been a huge transformation. For example, while I still firmly believe the best foods are predominantly whole, local, seasonal, and organic, I no longer look for confirmatory evidence of ill health in friends and loved ones who do not eat this way. Instead, I appreciate that health and resilience are available in a cornucopia of dietary choices.

I am not attached to being right. I'd rather be happy. I want to see thriving all around me, so I turn my gaze toward what I want to see. As I look for well-being, I notice it is popping up all over the place. I see the huge expansion of consciousness about buying locally from farmers' markets and community-supported agriculture. I watch movies like *The Economics of Happiness* and *I Am* succeed in reaching larger audiences. I appreciate the growing understanding of the connectedness of life, in diverse areas like Joel Salatin's and Michael Pollan's books, the Bioneers organization, and beekeeping journals. It is so interesting to me that this becomes easier and easier to do. It becomes more and more of a natural way to live. So in hearty response to Albert Einstein's quote that opened this chapter: "I choose the miraculous."

Tools for Transformation: Finding Miracles Everywhere

1. Synchronicity and miracles happen, often from fresh perspectives, openness, and allowing. *A Course in Miracles* teaches this as a spiritual truth, as does the delightful contemporary book *Pronoia Is the Antidote for Paranoia: How the Whole World Is Conspiring to Shower You with Blessings* by Rob Brezsny, though *Pronoia* is more playful. Both resources are full of insights and practical examples for shifting your perspective. "Pronoia" is an example of a consciousness-shifting new word we can include in our everyday speech.

2. Living life in a miraculous way requires letting yourself see a wider view of the world. In the next chapter, I go into much more detail about ways to expand perception. One way to enjoy more miracles in your life is to appreciate the many wonders that are already there for you.

   A fun tool for supporting your expansion is an "I love" writing exercise. Give yourself plenty of time for this tool—at least thirty minutes is important because you do not want to feel rushed. Get a notebook, a journal, or some paper. Write "I love" at the top of the page. Center and breathe, then start to think of all the things, people, places, and experiences you love. Begin with ones that are easy: your best memories, your kids or pets if you have them, your loved ones, features of nature, your favorite foods, music, places. There are no restrictions. Write down everything as it occurs to you. You can write anything from entire anecdotes to single words or names. Keep going, staying in that feeling of love, and let this flow. Have fun.

3. I once did this game for two hours, filling pages and pages of a journal. I felt euphoric by the end. The next few days were a study in delightful synchronicity as the people mentioned on my list phoned and emailed, and nature pulled out all the stops to remind me of the pleasures of alignment. See what is in store for you over the next days and hours when you play with this.

4. You can also try an eyes-open meditation tool where you stay in the present moment and see what you notice. This can be done in different ways. One is to just observe the flow, without writing anything down. Go to a lovely spot, indoors or outdoors, and get into a comfortable seated position. Again center and breathe, letting yourself relax deeply. Now observe everything you see, hear, smell, taste, and feel. Stay present. Colors, shapes, textures, light, pattern: Let your senses be as

full as they can. Breathe. You do not need to name the things you observe, even in your mind. Just stay open and let the impressions flow.

You can also try this while writing down your observations. Either way is fine, or try both and see which you like better. Stay in the present. If your thoughts drift, which they often do, relax, breathe, and bring yourself back to the present.

When I play this way I begin to get a great deal of kinesthetic information. My body feels electric, and my mind grows peacefully aware. See what you notice.

—CHAPTER FIFTEEN—

Communication

WHEN I AM ASKED TO teach some methods for discerning what elements of nature are saying, I begin with the most important step: accepting that communication is, in fact, possible. Before we get to *how* to perceive, it is essential to understand and allow the knowledge that what we can hear, see, comprehend, and interpret is real. The next, equally important step has to do with centering firmly in love and letting go of expectations. How to communicate is simple, once the reality of love is truly understood. Love will give direction to each of us regarding the most direct mode of interaction. Love is always communicating. How to connect resides entirely in the wisdom of the heart, guided by intuition. The mind interprets as the heart navigates.

From a space of love, we begin to notice that communication happens in many ways. Start with what you can directly sense, noticing the feelings elicited by your present-moment participation with nature. I have "prescribed" more time in nature on my patient instruction sheets for many years. Nature lifts our spirits. All we have to do is show up and be present in the moment. As we pay attention to the now moment we can be uplifted by a curious squirrel, shifting cloud formations, or a perfect morning glory translucent with sunlight. In wild terrains we might appreciate the howl of the wolf, feel the resonant croak of a bullfrog, or allow the profound and mysterious deep-sea song of whales to reverberate in us. Immeasurable amounts of sensory information are available to us. There is so much more to know as, led by our delight, we allow the whole of the present moment to fill our senses.

To foster communication, it is helpful to let go of analyzing our experiences as they occur. Release the internal running commentary on what is happening. Just be with it. Breathe. The less you catalogue your experiences and observations as they are happening, the more they will rearrange themselves in delightful and unexpected ways. Continue to breathe consciously. Insight resides in allowing our experiences to shape themselves, letting meaning emerge, rather than assigning it to thought categories already present.

Why is this so? Because how we already think about and understand things is not about the present moment. We tend to think about things based upon conclusions we have formed in the past. Those conclusions are a part of the past. They are about some old ways of thinking that we have been trained, or trained ourselves, to believe. But the communications of the natural world occur in the present. Everything happens *Now*. The past enters into the present only because we bring it along. We bring the past and even the potential future to the present by focusing upon it. Action and life is only ever in the now. In order to perceive anew, we must shift perspective, returning to a "beginner's mind." So breathe and relax, allowing yourself to come to the new experience as something fresh and alive.

In the Golden World it was clear to me that the only time that exists is Now; yet to have the experiences that form our lives, and the expansion that results from those experiences, we agree to exist in the dimension of linear time. These concepts may seem heady, or even a bit nutty. This is definitely not something the logical mind grasps easily. It is similar to a Zen koan or a Sufi tale—paradoxical questions or stories that bring you out of your tidy categorizations and into fresh, current, raw knowledge.

The brain is partially responsible for this paradox of understanding. The holistic, intuitive brain receives information, data, and perceptions hundreds of thousands of times more quickly than the analytical and logical brain can interpret them. In popular science lingo, this is categorized as "right and left brain" and in psychological terms is discussed as unconscious, subconscious, and conscious mind. In actuality, the human brain is more holographic, and all of this capacity is present everywhere. The analytical brain usually filters and selects what it will notice from the cornucopia of the brain's total awareness. It chooses based upon prior understanding. It is as if the brain is stating: "I will notice this but ignore that and will not bring it into conscious awareness." If that prior understanding excludes the immanence of nature or knowledge of our inner divinity, then our conscious access to that field of knowing is restricted.

The heart, on the other hand, innately understands the whole. The intelligence of the heart, with one-third as many neurons as the brain, helps us bypass our encrusted beliefs and allows fresh perspectives to flourish. Begin where you are, and move on from there. Stay detached from your interpretations of events. Just be present Now in order to hear, see, and understand: flutter of apple blossom, fragrance of lilac, enchantment of thyme, iridescent wing of dragonfly, sunbeams, sizzle of cicadas, moonbeams, moon shadows, cloud shadow, flickering firelight, tinkle of chimes, gentle sighs of a sleeping child. Olfactory, gustatory, emotional, sense of wonder, sense of wholeness, pattern of leaf and light, falling leaf anthems, dancing shadows, seed pop concertos, thump of acorns, crackling pine needles, softness of a baby's cheek. There are infinite varieties of information: jasmine fragrance flowing on a warm night breeze, color of flower, dance of bees, texture of air. Here a big gust that shakes many purple berries plunking to the ground, there a feeling of amazement, here a sense of knowing, there a flush of delight. Nature pens these words with me and a berry cluster bounces off my calf. Bamboo shimmers and whispers with each slight caress of the wind.

As we allow a wider field of perception we learn that nature will show us whatever we are expecting, whether or not we are consciously looking for it. Our life experience is a holographic representation of us, based on what we are emanating, also referred to as one's "vibration." Look around and notice what you see. Notice the things you notice. Breathe. Expand. Notice more. See if there is a theme within the things you tend to notice, and what types of things usually pass you by. This reveals more about you than it does about the state of the world. If you look around and see litter or traffic jams, observe the observer who notices. Then see what else you can notice. Can you see loveliness as well? It is definitely there. What is your dominant sense? Do you hear things, taste them, or smell them? Do you look up or down when you walk? Do you see patterns in the clouds and the flight of birds, or are you looking at the pavement beneath your feet? Do you see the beauty in the path? Do you first hear traffic noise, the song of the mockingbird, or a distant train whistle? Notice what meaning you extract from each of these, and then move on. We internally assign meaning to life experience but it is not absolute or externally generated. Meaning changes as we change.

Senses extend far beyond what is considered "normal" perception. As you pay more attention to what you notice, releasing assigned significance while remaining in the present moment, you will begin to develop tools for extension of the senses. Extrasensory perception is usually referred to in terms of the senses we already have. Clairaudience, for example, is extended hearing, while clairvoyance is extended seeing. "Extrasensory" perception is merely perceiving a bit more than we usually do.

Senses are extended from our ordinary human perspective. We know that other species sharing the planet have senses much keener than ours. Dogs can hear high-pitched whistles that are beyond most human hearing. Many animals—dogs, cats, and bears, to name a few— have a much more acute sense of smell than we do. They learn about occurrences in their environment by sniffing the wind and earth. Bees and other pollinating insects see light in the ultraviolet spectrum. We believe this shade appears to them in hues of a radiant blue. Many flowers capitalize on the extended vision of bees, displaying attractive markings in ultraviolet shades. Blossoms that to our eyes appear as ordinary "white" are like neon "bee highways" illuminating the road to nectar and pollen. Bats and dolphins navigate by echolocation, emitting a stream of high-frequency ultrasonic clicks up to two hundred thousand times per second. From the response wave of these clicks rebounding off natural forms, these animals easily locate prey and move about safely in darkness. A human child named Ben Underwood, blind since age two from a cancer in his eyes, taught himself to "see" by echolocation, astounding researchers.[1] Many birds navigate by connection to the magnetic core of the Earth. The mineral magnetite is found in their brains.

Interestingly, magnetite is also found in human brains. I wonder why? Do we also have a connection to the magnetic core of the Earth? Could it help us to navigate? Aboriginal people, many of whom are much closer to the natural world than "modern" people, can navigate in ways that seem magical to urban dwellers. Tribal people claim that they can feel the Earth. There is plenty of room here for further study within a science of love.

Vision in the animal kingdom can seem "extrasensory" from a human perspective. Soaring in the sky at a thousand feet, an eagle can spot a rabbit hopping in grass from a mile away. The compound eye of a simple housefly provides much more acute sight than our relatively simple human eyes.

Dolphins and whales communicate with one another, and probably other sea inhabitants, by means of sonar clicks and vibration. Most are not in audible range for human ears and require sensitive instruments to measure. Various insects and animals communicate through very rapid vibratory emissions. I have a beautiful CD called *God's Cricket Chorus*. The producers recorded cricket sounds, then slowed the recording down as if a normal cricket lifespan were as long as a human's. On average, crickets live only a few weeks, while humans live for about seventy-five years. These adjusted cricket sounds are truly breathtaking. The chorus sounds like angels singing.

In the natural world there are other, non-auditory modes of communication. Bees perform a complex dance to inform hive members of the location of a new patch of flowers, all in relationship to the angle of the sun. Animals, including humans, respond subconsciously to chemical messages such as pheromones. In fact, there are novel and costly pheromone perfumes available whose purpose is to make ordinary people seem extraordinarily attractive to others. And as we have seen, many bacteria navigate by chemotaxis, moving in response to chemical messages in the environment. Many of our own immune cells are mobilized in the same way.

It is astonishing that in spite of all this evidence of extended perception, humans have such a limited view of what is available to them. While they may accept that their dog is reading the newspaper of the neighborhood as she walks and sniffs the air and earth, there is little acknowledgement that we can receive information in these extended ways. Shamans talk of running with wolves and soaring with falcons. This is not simply a metaphor. It is an actual awareness. We truly can "borrow" the eyes of the eagle and the swiftness of the gazelle, if we can allow that sensitivity to exist within us. A view from the perspective of any animal, stone, or insect is available to us, if we are willing, allowing, and loving.

I know this first-hand, and you can too. I have had many experiences of sharing information with other beings. I have flown with dragonflies over glistening ponds and seen in all directions with their compound eyes. A dragonfly's field of vision is close to 360 degrees and they discern hues and vibrational ranges far beyond human perception. I have also relished consuming a delicious mouse while patrolling with a barn owl. Though eating a live mouse seems disgusting to my human self, while flying with the owl I savored each nuance of the experience. I am also aware of more primal experiences of knowing. I have been one with a drop of water falling into oceanic union, simultaneously sensing the joy of being at one with the ocean and the uniqueness of individuality as the droplet. I am aware of myself in the slow movement of crustal plates, as mountains rise and fall. I am aware of myself as the explosion of a supernova, hurtling the raw materials of new life out into the universe.

Those who have not yet opened their heart to the reality of these experiences could be missing out on a vital and delicious part of their birthright as humans. As one travels down these roads, the journey becomes easier. A shift of focus or consciousness can occur in a fraction of a second. It is simple to be the trembling blossom, beckoning to the hummingbird, and it is easy to hear the voice of deep-earth core layers communicated to a whale.

As we know ourselves in the ant, in the dolphin, in the cricket, or in the mycorrhizal community, we know something profoundly different about our nature than what we have been taught by our culture. We innately learn to respect and care for our natural world. For in caring for the air, the soil, and the sea, we nourish ourselves.

We already possess an abundance of easily accessible tools for enhanced communication. Our dreams are one such vehicle. The ancient Egyptians held the information transmitted through dreams in high regard, believing that dream-state messages could offer cures for waking illnesses. The "dreaming prophet" Edgar Cayce believed likewise, as did many of his devotees who consulted him while he was in the dream state for cures to their ailments. Many of these treatments were highly effective. In the Bible, Joel 2:28, it is written, "I will pour out my Spirit upon all people. Your sons and daughters will prophesy. Your old men will dream dreams, and your young men will see visions."

Certain indigenous people have highly coherent dreams, such as the dreamtime of Aboriginal Australians. Some of these cultures find more value from dream reality than waking reality. In his book *The Four Agreements*, Toltec shaman don Miguel Ruiz explains that all life is a dream. There is a waking dream and a sleeping dream.

I receive profound insights from my dreams. The emotional content of my dreams gives me a bead on feelings I may be either suppressing or glossing over in daily life. As a tool, dreams can remind us of familiar and overlooked patterns in our lives. In my life's journey, I notice that the universe loves a joke and a pun, and humor shows up a lot in my dreams. Often I get clarifying dream messages that are humorous or silly. For example, while writing, I had been working with my own fears about theft and security. I am writing a number of books, and they are all saved on this one little portable computer. I had been practicing letting go of my fears by centering in my heart, just as I teach patients and discuss throughout this book. Yet I continued to be bothered by niggling fears and insecurities, and would often carry my computer with me in a large handbag rather than leave it at home or in my car trunk.

As I headed toward a place of peace and allowing, I dreamt that I was traveling with friends and we were crossing the border into Mexico. My friends were unencumbered but I was carrying a large suitcase. It had wheels but was unwieldy. Wherever we went—restaurants, shops, or the beach—I had to maneuver this suitcase even though there was no need for it in any of those places. My friends had left their bags at the hotel, but I continued to carry mine along with me. I woke up wondering why in the world am I carrying around all this baggage, and I was truly amused by the concreteness of the metaphor of the dream.

A few nights later I dreamt that I was packing in order to move to a new home. I had already packed all that I wanted and needed; this was collected in several trunks. But there remained a lot of "stuff" including half-used cleaning products, trinkets that I no longer used or enjoyed, and clothing that no longer fit. And, to cap it off, while packing I was spending time with a man with whom I'd had a brief relationship thirty years before and was, once again, finding it unsatisfying. I began to listlessly pack these left-over items, but then thankfully awoke and came to the realization that I no longer needed to carry any of this along with me. The thoughts and attitudes about past relationships, the old clothes, were like old skins—they were baggage I could easily shed. I realized that my fears about security and possessions came from outdated beliefs. There was no need to pack them up and cart them along with me. As a result, it became easier to focus upon what I truly did want to carry forward with me, things that were meaningful and nourishing. I was inspired to upload my books to a couple of zip drives and began to feel secure about leaving the computer at home. My shoulders relaxed.

There are many places one can go to learn about developing greater skills at extending perception. The Monroe Institute, also called TMI—located about an hour from Charlottesville, Virginia—is a nondenominational, non-profit institute dedicated to expanding human potential. Exploring consciousness is their bread and butter. Having attended many of their programs, I can whole-heartedly recommend them.

The founder, Robert Monroe, was a visionary and intrepid explorer of inner space and consciousness. Monroe was a writer, producer, and director of a number of popular radio programs. Bob, as people who study at the institute affectionately know him, had a chronic problem with insomnia. He was also fascinated by the idea of learning during sleep. Being familiar with radio and the power of sound, he began experimenting in the 1950s with various tones and frequencies to try to auditorily stimulate the brain-wave pattern of deep sleep. These early experiments did not immediately produce the desired results: Monroe found that his sleep did not improve with the use of the tones—in fact, he developed a persistent humming sensation throughout his body, noticeable especially when falling asleep. Even when he abandoned the auditory inputs for a while, the weird humming sensations continued to occur frequently, especially just as he was falling asleep.

A few months into this experiment, Monroe "popped" out of his body while drifting off to sleep. He felt fully awake and conscious, yet found himself floating above the sleeping forms of his physical body and that of his wife. The first time it unnerved him, yet he quickly became intrigued by what was happening. He was bolstered by the enthusiasm of his physician, in whom he confided what he was experiencing. After ruling out a brain tumor or other serious health problem, this wise doctor did not send Monroe for lengthy psychotherapy—he offered him a clean bill of health and encouraged him to continue to explore the phenomenon.[2]

This is exactly what Monroe did. He wrote three fascinating books about his adventures. After some exploration, Bob Monroe coined the now-popular term "out-of-body experience," or OBE. All three of his books, the first of which is *Journeys Out of Body*, published in 1971, are still in print. He continued OBE journeys for the remainder of his life. Bob resumed investigating frequencies and tones and developed a method called Hemi-Sync®, or hemispheric synchronization.[3]

Hemi-Sync® technology blends tones to assist perception in various ways. Certain tonal combinations support alertness and concentration; others enhance deep meditation. Monroe and his co-explorers eventually developed combinations to support the deep and refreshing sleep that he sought. The method works well, even with the deaf, since the vibrations are transmitted by bone conduction. As Bob grew more comfortable with the terrain of non-physical reality, he recognized a growing need to assist others to have and understand these experiences. Some people already had experienced similar phenomena but were afraid and wanted some reassurance and guidance. Others wanted the experiences but had no idea how to achieve them. Hence the Monroe Institute was born. Monroe and a group of explorers of inner space worked out tone combinations that easily elicited profound altered states of consciousness without drugs. I affectionately consider Bob Monroe to have been one of the first techno-shaman pioneers. An interesting thing, which they will explain to you at the Monroe Institute, is that utilizing the Hemi-Sync® exercises can be compared to putting training wheels on a bicycle. They are simply tools to help people access their innate capacities.

Tools for Transformation

1. Try working with dreams as an exercise in extending your communication abilities. Dreams are best recorded when they are fresh, immediately upon awakening. Keep a bedside dream journal and write down dreams as soon as you wake up. Analyzing their content comes later. Consider participating in a dream group with friends or attending a dream workshop or conference.

2. Since dreams are profoundly personal, I encourage you not to get stuck in rigid interpretations. There is no simple correlation between dream images and life details. There are dream books out there that will purport to tell you exactly what each dream image symbolizes. While this may apply with certain archetypal images, interpreting in this way is akin to utilizing only one layer of interpretation. Instead, notice first how your dreams feel to you. Are they peaceful, unsettling, scary, or funny? The emotional content of dreams, especially how they feel to you upon awakening, can tell you a lot about the dominant themes of your current life. So write the feelings you awaken with down in your dream journal, perhaps in a separate column, alongside the storyline and images. Did different dreams or dream segments feel different to you?

3. Images can also be helpful, but remember that any meaning assigned should feel correct to you and not just be someone else's blanket interpretation. At times, dream images can reconstruct recent events in a novel way, allowing new insights about an existing situation. As you become more comfortable

working with dreams, you might directly request dream insights about pertinent issues you are trying to resolve, before you slumber.

4. Once you have written down all the basic details, analyze them in a way that feels congruent to you. Do any of the emotions or images feel familiar to you from recent life experiences? Notice if there are any resonances with current life themes. How might your subconscious be communicating new insights to you about your predominant state of focus?

5. If your dreams are disturbing, don't worry! There is useful information you can glean. You subconscious mind is trying to get through to your conscious mind. Is some situation in your life causing similar feelings? If so, can you shift how you are looking at it?

6. If dreams feel happy, exhilarating, or profound, enjoy the ride. Can you amplify those feelings? Find congruence between your waking-life actions that elicit similar joyous emotions in the dream states. These feelings show you when are on a track harmonious with your soul's current purpose. These are avenues worthy of greater exploration and development in your daily life.

—CHAPTER SIXTEEN—

Visions of a Seer

WHILE WRITING THIS BOOK I often found myself humming the words "give yourself to love" from the hauntingly lovely song by the late Kate Wolf. Love nourishes every fiber of our being. In living the ways of love, we consciously contribute our benevolent legacy to the world around us. My dream of the future is that this understanding becomes more widespread. I imagine a maturation of humanity in which love, gentleness, and kindness become "cool" because they reflect the best in us. I am excited to think of the cultural shifts available to humanity as our little mirror neurons reflect a worldview of integrity, love, trust, possibilities, acceptance, and well-being. I imagine a world filled with the understanding that each life has meaning and purpose. A comprehension of our interconnectedness grows. We are part of a greater whole that includes humanity, all living things, inanimate matter, and non-physical reality. I choose to dream this world into being, joining with all who dream and see.

You might have picked up this book because you seek a new understanding of health that is heart-centered and honors spirit. Perhaps you are a scientist, and from the first mention of dissection of a live frog you felt some uneasiness, some knowledge that there must be a different, kinder way to study life. Maybe you garden and love to nurture growing things, or you delight in sitting or walking in nature. I believe we are here because the planet, and consciousness itself, is calling to us—calling patients, physicians, scientists, students, and dreamers alike to form loving relationships, to awaken to the interrelated whole of who we are, and we are starting to hear its voice.

We are at an important crossroads. Each of us can make a difference in shifting the winds and defining the course of the new model that is now emerging. Do not underestimate what you can accomplish as you come into harmonious relationship with your true self and with the natural world. Positive focus accomplishes miracles. Dare to dream, and to listen. The future is in our hands.

I have heard people say, "The Earth is angry with us, it wants us gone." I believe nothing is further from the truth. Earth's natural world is always singing to the universe of a new balance, born of a motion toward ever-greater love. This new balance is not anti-human. We know that we are a part of nature and a part of the cumulative chorus. The voice of nature is not asking for our destruction. Instead, it is gently coaxing our cooperation into consciousness. Nature is weaving a pattern of deeper understanding and interconnectedness into the fibers of our being. Our present-moment focus determines whether we see externally what is already in our hearts, but more and more of us are recognizing the truth of our spiritual essence and contemplating its astounding ramifications for physical life.

In our deepest wonderings, we ask many questions. Why are we here? What is my role? What is the substance of physical reality? What are we made of? How are we all connected? Both science and spirituality attempt to answer these questions. In the ancient times it was said, "All roads lead to Rome." The answer of diverse spiritual traditions is that all roads, all paths lead home, and home is love.

The founding saint of the Sikh faith, Guru Nanak, a fifteenth-century mystic, said, "There is no Hindu, there is no Muslim." His meaning is the same as that of the contemporary Hindu teacher Ramana Maharshi's simple statement: "There are no others." There is only divinity at the heart of each of us. Our dichotomizations are our own creation, which become our crosses to bear until we allow them to fall away. They become our life challenges and our health problems. The big knotty dichotomizations that many of us share become societal problems.

Materialistic science answers the question, "What is the substance of physical reality?" by breaking matter down into smaller and smaller particles. What remains after all these particles are discovered? Will they ever all be discovered? Yes, there are atoms, which are made up of subatomic particles: quarks, hadrons, etc. But what are these composed of? From the level of quantum physics, they are the elusive descriptor/premise "energy" that has still not been characterized. Physicist Werner Heisenberg referred to elementary particles as "the idea of matter."[1] A new particle that may require physicists to rethink their standard model of particle physics was discovered at Fermi labs on April 6, 2011.[2,3] Quantum physics explains simply that matter is inextricably related to energy. $E=MC^2$. What appears solid is only a dancing extension of a universal energy source. But this still begs the question, what is energy?

Materialistic science without a spiritual underpinning is a flat earth. It is a model that cannot contain the whole of what we now know. When a photon is in superposition, before the presence of an observer, does it even exist in physical reality? If not, then physical reality is entirely determined by the mind of the observer.

In a 1979 *Scientific American* article, physicist Bernard d'Espagnat observed, "The doctrine that the world is made up of objects whose existence is independent of human consciousness turns out to be in conflict with quantum mechanics and the facts established by experiment."[4] A provocative BBC program aired in 2011 argued that reality exists in a purely mathematical framework.[5] Spiritual adepts throughout the ages have explained that reality exists within consciousness, not separate from it. We are now witnessing the birth of a broader science to "prove" it. Ultimately, all that we see, all that we experience, all that we are—is in the mind of God, or divinity, or source, or spirit. Pick your favorite term. We are spiritual beings living a physical reality that is spiritual by its very nature. As the stuff of divinity, we are endlessly free to create and play and choose within our playground of physical reality. But the game can be so much more fun when we know who we really are.

The German Christian mystic Rudolf Steiner said, "Matter is condensed light." Abraham says, "Matter is extended thought." On a personal out-of-body journey, I asked my guides about the composition of physical reality and was answered not with words, but with a vision. I saw brilliant light coming into material reality as through a membrane. Physical-to-be substance was nestled, snuggly and lovingly, in this membrane-like material that hovers between the worlds. All below it, beside it, and above it is composed of a glistening that is only one substance, both non-physical and physical, and that is love. The "matter" parts of us are just nestled bits of condensation/expansion of the same material that holds it all together. Infusing the tiniest particles, the hadrons, the quarks, and the elusive Higgs boson, there is love and consciousness of love. The Earth, the Solar System, the Milky Way galaxy, the known Universe, and the suspected multiverse are all made of the same substance: Love. The answers to all the questions are the same. Energy=thought=light=love.

Love animates all matter and all life. You know this love in your heart. You know this when you look at wholeness that has just come forth from love and is still aware of its nestled nature: a new baby, a puppy, a kitten, and the first cotyledons of a sprouting seed. All of these reach naturally for the light. You know this when you see the rays of the sun shining out from behind a cloud, or when you observe the streaming of light in a forest. It is in the song of the bullfrog, the patter of raindrops, and the fragrance of roses. You know love as you settle into the simple ease of your own breath. We are renewed with each breath. Our breathing marks the movement of eternity into time.

Who are we? We are creatures of love. What is the world? It is the body of love, the fabric of love. Nothing is sacred or profane, except in our own minds. We are only beginning, as a society, to factor the perspective of love into scientific inquiry. I certainly do not claim to have all the answers, and new questions constantly emerge.

Will there be new scientific principles and laws that factor in love? Yes, certainly, but they are likely to be related to understanding the nature of consciousness, quite different laws than those that Newton and mechanistic scientists relied upon. The nature of the universe, the cosmos, and our physical earthly existence is vastly different than they understood. They looked at a small fragment and called it whole. Life and physical existence is meaningful, not mechanistic. It is closer to miraculous.

As I mention throughout this book, I sometimes hear fear-based words that demonize certain organisms. Many people have an attitude that bacteria, fungi, spirochetes, and viruses as well as rats, ants, and mosquitoes are at best opportunistic, and at their worst malevolently out to get us. Nothing could be further from the truth, and I hope through reading what I have offered here, you now have a sense of this too. If we believe the Universe is intelligent, and we understand that love underlies all reality, then we can begin to accept that microbes, a part of "all reality," are also part of that love.

As eternal beings, no real harm may come to us. All-that-is wishes us well, loves us deeply and unconditionally, for we are each a part, a spoke, a ray, a sunbeam of all-that-is. We are light. The purpose of life is greater love. The microbial world, like the animal, plant, and insect kingdoms, cares deeply about us. Though each member of the microbial world is on its own unique trajectory toward its own particular crystallization of greater love, it knows us only in the space of love. It only offers what everything else in creation offers—a magic mirror of the sum our thoughts and beliefs in this now moment.

If there is harm, it is we who do apparent harm to ourselves. Our apparent self-injury is mirrored to us by other beings, including microorganisms. I emphasize the word "apparent" here because, in time, short or long, we all come into knowledge of the law of love. Microorganisms, mice, breezes, and thunderstorms intersect with us merely as cooperative players in our individual and collective dramatic dreams.

Love or fear is our ultimate choice. To grow in enlightenment is to accept the "other" as self. Our current science, though limited and compartmentalized, is now showing us, literally, that the narrow ways we think of ourselves are not correct. Everything interconnects. Elementary particles are entangled, perpetually connected despite distance between them. In fact, with entanglement, distance is meaningless. Mathematical physicist Roger Penrose explained: "Quantum entanglement is a very strange type of thing. It is somewhere between objects being separate and being in communication with each other."[6] Quantum entanglement explains a wider view of how reality works. It provides a framework for a holographic understanding of physical existence.

In a hologram, every part reflects and displays the whole. In his book *The Holographic Universe* author Michael Talbot explains how quantum science suggests that all of what we perceive as solid physical reality is actually a holographic image projection of a greater reality that exists beyond the bounds of time and space. This is just as Plato discussed more than twenty-five hundred years ago in the allegory of the cave.[7] In his allegory, we live as if we are prisoners in a dark cave—we see and hear shadows and echoes made by unseen objects, and believe the reflected images are all that is. But true reality is infinitely more complex and vibrant.

The whole is always greater than the sum of its parts. Dissection into parts—removing isolated individuals from the whole, from community—gives no real information about the majesty of who we really are. Instead it leads us down a blind alley where we "know more and more about less and less, until we know everything about nothing."

If there are more bacteria in and on us than cells of our "own" bodies, then who are we? If there are billions of viruses dormant in our system at any given time, and our cells decide whether and when to activate them, then who are we? What are we creating? Who is doing the creating? Can we trust the "others" who we are? Can we trust our own cells? Each of our cells has formerly independent organisms, the mitochondria, running the show of energy production. Each cell and each organ has its own bit of consciousness, its own tropism toward greater love. So who are we in this community, in this chorus of life? Who is the "I" here? Can we trust the breath that moves us into time? Can we trust the life force that animates us? Can we trust the center, the heart?

I understand as truth Einstein's eloquent statement, "God does not play dice with the universe." Existence is meaningful. The missing piece, which Einstein did not state, is our own divinity, and the divinity of all physical and non-physical existence. God does not play dice with the universe because we are in and of God. That is the mystical understanding of unity, and therein is the ability each of us has to play in the fields of the divine. Understanding that life is meaningful, we can create thriving health in our body and harmony in our world.

Less than five hundred years ago a deal was made in Europe. It was a good deal at the time. The seventeenth-century churches, both Catholic and Protestant, had a stranglehold on information. Dominant religious institutions did not accept our individual inner divinity. They wanted to mediate between the divine and our consciousness. The fresh air of science supplanted all of this. It was an evolutionary change, and the early understanding of Darwin's scientific observations contributed to our mind's liberation. The Renaissance of scientific understanding allowed humanity greater freedom. Unhampered independent and creative thought flourished. But now we have taken that rich vein of exploration to a logical conclusion. We are ready for an understanding of the power of consciousness, ready to understand that we are all connected at deep and basic levels, ready to know that each of us is an expression of the divine, and each of us can personally communicate with that greater sphere of knowing.

There is no need to decry the expansion of consciousness that brought us to this new threshold of awareness. Overly mechanistic, it has merely run its course, and consciousness is making way for the new, the next expansion. I tell my patients as they are working through their problems, "When this pattern began, it was functional. It was the best choice at the time. But like an old overcoat, the one you loved when you were six, that was warm and snuggly then—it is way too tight now." Five hundred years ago, even two hundred years ago, a science of mechanistic materialism was a good choice, but now it no longer fits who we have become and what we know.

Contemporary science and its child, modern medicine, often ignore who we really are. Each of us creates ourselves, creates our lived reality. There is a science to this. But if we leave out the most important data points—that our experience of the universe is subjective, that we are divine spiritual beings in a sacred universe composed of love, that we are creators, and that the Law of Attraction is how things get matched up—then we are left with a science that is woefully incomplete.

I am thrilled by the prospect of a science that is loving, cooperative, whole, and alive; a science that recognizes and honors the love that underlies the substance of physical reality. This is the only science that will carry us physically to the stars, to other universes, and to the infinity of the love in our own hearts.

What then, does a new medicine based on love look and feel like? It includes trust, integrity, respect, humor, beauty, and joy. It honors the heart and nature. It is life-affirming, creative, and fun. But these are all abstract concepts and there is much concrete understanding that is being born of new science. The science of love includes the science of expanding consciousness, psi phenomena, and cooperative communication with nature.

Long term, there will be fundamental change in how we understand our bodies, and in what we call "health care." There are many roads that can get us there, with many pragmatic stops along the way. Changes will be seen at every level: personal, community, and society.

This is already underway. Initially, in practical terms, we will see exploration and adoption of more environmentally friendly technologies, like thermographic imaging, that create no nuclear waste. Health insurance will cover preventive and rebalancing "alternative" remedies like acupuncture, manual osteopathy, and chiropractic. There will be continued examination of the real costs of medicine, with an eventual understanding that herbs and homeopathic remedies are significantly less costly, more harmonious with our physiology, and much more environmentally sound than most pharmaceuticals. In Cuba, since the U.S. embargo, there has been a flourishing of green medicine. Clinics grow herbs. People in Cuba are healthy even though their medical system, per capita, costs only a fraction of our current one.

Nature, the environment, and nutrition will be factored in as costs in health care debates. As we understand that we are interrelated and intertwined, we will understand that we cannot have healthy food without healthy soil. We cannot have healthy bodies without healthy oceans, seas, and rivers or without a healthy vibrant atmosphere. We will promote diverse and vigorous colonies of soil microbes in our agriculture, knowing that the foods grown in them will be much richer in nutrients, and will support our own normal flora as well. We will protect the waters of our planet, for they are the life force of our own bodies. We will cease to use technologies that poison the atmosphere, recognizing that the Earth's atmosphere is its lungs, and therefore it is our lungs. Eventually we will appreciate the thriving of the soil and the seas, as living beings, for their own sake. As we appreciate health in one arena we more easily celebrate it through the whole. We will do this by making personal choices regarding how we eat, how we shop, and what we feel we need to consume.

There will be changes in agriculture. We will look more at solutions like permaculture and grass-based agriculture. We will have smaller local farms that support thriving communities. Agriculture will be organic. We are already rediscovering simple, safe, and marvelously effective sources of enriching our soils, such as use of very dilute sea-water and extremely dilute sea salt.[8] Shallow seas are believed to have once covered almost the entire surface of the planet, forming the mineral structure of our soils. The mineral composition of seawater is virtually identical to that of the earth-dwelling beings that the oceans sustain. Simple dilute seawater may be the perfect non-toxic, sustainable fertilizer for enlivening soil.

We will come to gladly pay the real costs of nutritious foods, rather than believing we are getting a bargain by consuming ersatz cheap food. There will be more dietary advice not related to a corporate agenda, more examination of traditional food ways. Our minds and bodies will thrive. All of this is underway. Farmers' markets that bring consumers local, organic, and sustainably grown nutritious foods are popping up all over the place. In fact, a new one opened a few weeks ago, literally one block from my office. These same markets bring farmers and farming communities a dignified, wholesome, and sustainable lifestyle.

We will discontinue energy production methods, like nuclear energy, that inevitably create health damage through generating waste. We will move on to safe and sustainable forms of energy, because we must. Research in renewable energy sources—geothermal, solar, hydroelectric, and wind—is expanding and will continue to grow. Even cold fusion, once ridiculed as an impossibility, appears very likely as a near-term reality. Recent experiments at the University of Bologna in Italy demonstrate that much more energy is generated by a small cold-fusion reactor developed there than is consumed.[9] The energy is produced safely, with no resultant nuclear waste.[10] Many investigators are looking at zero-point energy and other sustainable and safe technologies that almost sound like science fiction but may be quite viable and right around the corner.

As individuals and as societies, we will once again pay attention to the effects of our current choices on the next seven generations, and beyond. For if we are all one, then we are our future generations. In understanding our unity, we understand that caring for one another, the earth, plants, animals, and microbes is indeed caring for ourselves.

We will continue to mature in caring for ourselves. We will grow in the understanding that our physical health relates to our emotional health and inner well-being. Agendas that are financially profitable for a very few while fragmenting communities or unbalancing the environment will no longer seem appealing to anyone, even to the few who might "profit." Mutual aid and compassion will be understood as healthy choices for all of us.

Technologically, what does this mean? There will be medical breakthroughs and insights. These may look like the small hand-held biofeedback device called Scenar™, developed in Russia for their space program that has wide application for healing a variety of ailments. It may look like growing mushrooms and working cooperatively with plants in bioremediation to purify water and clean up toxic wastes created within the old paradigm. It may look like research into health benefits of color and light, or gentle but deep healing based on sound and tone.

There will be more honing and sharing of ancient healing wisdom like Ayurveda and Traditional Chinese Medicine and assistive technologies to enhance them. There will be assistance from nature in a variety of ways, including utilizing gentle tools like flower essences and spagyric medicines, and dialogue with bacteria and fungi about balancing health.

There will be more practitioners who look at the bigger picture. Self-reflection and rebalancing tools like meditation, Qi gung, aikido, and yoga will continue to grow in popularity. Complementary and alternative medicine is a huge and expanding segment of the health care market. Currently one-third to two-thirds of Americans seeking medical treatment utilize some complementary and alternative medical treatments.[11] Fifty years ago, only a tiny fraction of the population used these types of treatments, and even thirty years ago they were rarely employed. Today mind-body techniques, acupuncture, homeopathy, and manual techniques like craniosacral and chiropractic have become mainstream. More than fifty percent of people who use these therapies are not ill but work with them to prevent illness.[12]

More patients will go to the doctor to be soothed and to feel more empowered about the available choices. There will be more and more clean medicines and healing tools, made in partnership with nature, that are in harmony with the planet. We are learning to listen to our hearts. There will be rich soils, biodiversity, and nutritious foods. There will be cooperation. There will be technology, but of a sort that harmonizes with the natural world. Because of this, there will be great beauty.

Perhaps one day the CDC will stand for Centers for Disease Communication. Perhaps virologists will be people who communicate with viruses, and bacteriologists will talk with bacteria in their own language, much as artist Anna Dumitriu does. While some of this seems playfully magical to our present way of thinking, remember that airplanes, cell phones, television, and moon walks were flights of fantasy a mere century ago. I met a physicist at the Monroe Institute who uses the information he collects during out-of-body journeys to design his new experiments. He has been quite successful and has even won awards for his research, though he is very private about the exploration journeys. Magic is merely that which we do not currently comprehend.

Eventually, I believe, the new medicine may look like no medicine at all. No sickness need come to us, though this will be a journey of the evolution of human consciousness with many interesting stops along the way. We can eventually spend our time on more and more individual and cooperative creative endeavors. Visionaries have seen us expanding into a galactic community, as full citizens, with telepathic communication with enlightened beings becoming commonplace.

This project started out as a book about the tiniest life forms and a way of imagining a different, more loving, and more harmonious relationship with them than the one projected by "modern" industrial scientific thought. While it is still that, it has grown to something much bigger in the writing. I know it is our future, because some of us are already there. We can live as the divine beings we are, with the loving cooperation of a divine universe that we also are. Let's imagine together the loving, glorious co-creation that is possible. So it is with profound appreciation to the tiny and tremendous worlds which inspire me that I offer this ancient new perspective.

TOOLS FOR TRANSFORMATION: WAVES OF LOVE

1. Love waves are a simple but powerful tool for supporting the Earth and transforming consciousness. The idea initially came from my inner guidance during a meditation retreat, and it has been supported by a series of visions I have had over the past four years. I was also influenced by Dean Radin's research findings on coherence in random-number generators when people focus together (so far, usually on some negative world event), and Joseph Chilton Pearce's discussion of the significance of the toroidal-shaped electromagnetic fields of the Earth.

   I had been musing about all the negative focus we have in regard to the planet. Our worries about "global warming" and pollution seemed misplaced—not because of the "reality" or lack of it for these concerns, but because I know, as I have discussed in this book, that the discoveries of leading-edge physics confirm the essential wisdom of many profound spiritual teachings. The essence of these teachings is that we are interconnected, and our thoughts and focus mold and influence what we believe to be objective reality. I wondered what might happen if large groups of people intentionally focused together positively and with love?

Simply stated: we are powerful creators, and it is our focus that creates our experience both individually and collectively. So having a lot of people worrying about the well-being of our planet, or life on Earth, is not beneficial for any of us. Focusing together on well-being can powerfully catalyze positive change for the Earth as well as for society.

Look inside yourself. How many choices do you make personally based on fear and how many based on love? What are the outcomes of these choices? I have noticed that fear-based choices have never led to anything I really wanted. I have come to realize that in every instance as I choose love, I flourish, my joy increases, and the world around me looks more like an image of that love.

2. It occurred to me that it would be easy to focus together positively, and that the final exercise of this book would be a perfect place to introduce this visionary exercise. Group focus would best be done at significant, simple-to-remember points of the year. The natural compass of the year, observed in solstices and equinoxes, links us with past and future generations and with the cycles and seasons of the planet. It is a perfect time frame for these waves.

3. The essence of the wave project is this: We surround the Earth with our positive thoughts, ideas, visions, and vibrations at least four times per year, forming a coherent wave of love and well-being that encircles the planet. By joining together at specific times, in meditation, prayer, and appreciation, we consciously create Waves of Love that travel and surround the Earth with good and coherent thoughts and emotions. While participating, we visualize our positive images of what we love best about life on Earth and human civilization, along with our deepest hopes and aspirations for our future and the future of our planet. We see our individual and collective selves

thriving. We envision understanding and peace growing on our planet.

4. Love Waves are an opportunity for us as individuals to dream together. The Love Waves are an invitation to participate in the co-creation of a glorious vision for ourselves, and for our beloved home planet. Ultimately, they are for the benefit of all consciousness.

5. Our images do not need to be visual images, because not all of us are visual. Impressions, feelings, sounds, words, and sensations are all images, since every image is simply an electromagnetic vibration. What we call physical reality is created by our collective thoughts. Our individual reality relates to our personal thoughts, while the larger reality relates to thoughts of humanity. Thoughts, a form of vibration, exist as electromagnetic energy. They are measurable, via EEG and other instrumentation. Once generated, thought wave/particles are infinite.

6. Our emotions inform us as to whether our creations will feel good to us when they arrive. Emotions are one way that higher guidance communicates with us. If we have good-feeling emotions—if our vision makes us excited, happy, joyous, or even blissful—then we are heading to manifestations that we will love. But if our visions cause anxiety, worry, or feelings of uneasiness, then we are pointing ourselves to creation of something that we do not really want. I have worked with these principles for many years, with clear and tangible results. In every situation that we face personally or as a society, we always have a choice about how to feel, and this choice determines our actions. The choice can be summarized as love versus fear.

7. The application of these basic concepts on a global scale equals the Love Wave. So whatever we send out is best sent from love. It should feel good, high, happy, joyous, and wonderful.

As we transmit the beam, we receive the beam, in equal measure. In the eloquent words of Lennon/McCartney, "… And in the end, the love you take is equal to the love you make."

8. The more we participate in positive activism like the Love Waves, the more the vision expands. The wave blankets the Earth with "good vibrations," with love, harmony, light, and well-being. The wave includes as many people as are inspired by this vision.

   In your visions and imaginings, be sure to see good for yourself, and for others as well as the planet. We are all good, all worthy, all loved by our creator, by source, by all-that-is, by the universe, by ultimate reality, however we understand this to be. If you want greater peace of mind, more love, better relationships, and greater prosperity, understand that we are holographic projections of the infinite, and there is no limit to the abundance of well-being available in our world, so go ahead and see good for yourself and others in your visions. Do any of this any time you feel inspired!

9. The Love Wave is non-denominational. There is no need to identify with a particular faith, or you can identify with any faith. The Wave grows as it keeps circling the globe, and greater love, greater mutual understanding, and greater harmony will ensue.

   Ideally, throughout the day, there will be people meditating at every moment, focusing on the well-being of the planet, our visions of harmony, joy, cooperation, and appreciation of one another, as well as our love for all beings of this world: humans, animals, insects, and microbes. Also, we might feel and express appreciation for all the material things that are in our world: water, earth, air, fire, minerals, buildings, roads, bridges, and electricity. The list can go on forever. Thus we blanket the Earth with feelings of love and good will.

10. Guided meditation is one possibility for participation in the Waves of Love. These can enhance our focus. I am including the text of one sample meditation in the appendix.

Feel free to use the meditation I provide, or one of your own. Put a reminder on your calendar and tune in. We are not focusing on what some people think is broken or wrong, or our worries, because we want to attract energy to what we want, by positive focus. Instead focus on our lives and the world, as we love to see her, and notice what is working well. See what is positive in the world around you. Look around and consider all the things that you love as your contribution to the greater good on a particular day. Visualize or imagine things getting better and better, with more and more harmony circulating our planet, more people and other beings living in friendship, compassion, and optimism. What would that feel like to you? Feel those feelings now.

Consciousness is shifting. In our consciousness, we can experience the tiniest subatomic particle, or we can hold the flow of a whole galaxy. The more we create through love and see love, the easier it will be to see our visions manifesting on the physical plane. Watch for this happening more and more!

Appendix

Sample Guided Meditation

Listen to me read this on the website www.worldlovewaves.com (for free, including a free downloadable podcast), or read and record it yourself, or just do your own thing!

Have you ever seen a lake so placid that it perfectly reflects the sky above and the scenery surrounding it? Deep inside each of us is stillness, an inner knowing, and a place of inner peace. Divinity reflects itself in our inner stillness. Let's breathe and relax and go to that place of inner stillness now.

Breathe in love. Breathe it in to your heart. Breathe out love. See it swirl around you.

Imagine that Earth is a planet known throughout the universe for its magnificent beauty and diversity. Think of a beautiful, peaceful place that you love. This may be by the ocean, in the mountains, or in a placid meadow. It may be in your village or your backyard. Feel the serenity there.

Now think about something or someone you love. This can be your child, your parent, your spouse, a mentor, or a friend. It can be an animal, a pet, or a natural area such as a waterfall or a mountain. Feel the love you have. Breathe out the love you feel and breathe it back inside yourself.

Expand the love that you feel. Send it to your body. Appreciate and love your body—every cell, every organ, and every limb. Your body is wonderful and miraculous. Rest in the love and remember how it feels.

Now send this love to your community, town, or city. Breathe it out to everyone and everything you know, and breathe it back in from them.

Send the love to your whole region; see health in the people, in the soil, in the waters. Send love to the microbes, the insects, the plants, and the animals. Breathe love to the atmosphere and breathe it back.

Send love to and through the Earth. Breathe love into the core of the Earth, and breathe back the love that is there. See your feet as roots planted firmly and deeply in nourishing soil. Feel the warmth of the earth, feel the love of the sun pouring light upon you, and feel the healthy mycelia nourishing your root tips.

Think of water: of streams, rain, rivers, brooks, lakes, oceans, humidity. Send your love to the water of the Earth and receive love back. Think of sea creatures: whales, dolphins, fish, coral reefs, jellyfish, seaweeds, the myriad of life that teems in our oceans, from the single-celled phytoplankton to the immense and profound blue whale. Send your appreciation to the beings of the ocean, to the ocean currents, to the tides, to the seashore, and receive love and appreciation in return. Think of the beach, the serenity of the tides; think of the tides in our own bodies, and the waters in all life. Send your love. See the perfection. See the beauty. Know that all is well.

Now think of air, of fragrance, wind, breezes, of the blanket of our atmosphere, of air currents that buoy the birds and the clouds. Think of air, of its constituent elements: nitrogen, oxygen, carbon dioxide, and many other gases in small amounts—methane, helium, hydrogen, argon—and how perfectly the composition of this atmosphere is for us and for other beings. We breathe in air and our lungs take in oxygen, we exhale and release carbon dioxide. The plants inhale carbon dioxide and exhale oxygen in a timeless dance of love. See the air crisp and clean, love the atmosphere, and love its well-being. Appreciate. Take a deep breath. Breathe in the love and breathe it back out.

Now, think of the earth, the soils, the mycorrhizae extending under vast regions, the types of earth: rocks, sand, metals, and minerals. The rocks know the longevity of well-being. Appreciate the minerals in our bodies, the iron at the center of each molecule of hemoglobin, the calcium, magnesium, silica, and phosphorus in our bones. Think of the beauty of crystals. Imagine a crystal cave, amplifying your love. Breathe.

Think of the fire of the sun that warms us and the fire of metabolism that nourishes each cell. Think of the fire of distant stars that became the elements of our bodies. Breathe love to all of them and breathe it back.

Surround the Earth with love. Now extend the love you feel to the entire universe. Breathe in love, breathe out love. Breathe in peace, breathe out peace. Enjoy the feelings you have created. Relax. The work you have done is very real and very powerful. Thank yourself for participating in our majestic, conscious co-creation.

Bibliography and Resources

Adas, Michael. *Machines as the Measure of Men: Science, Technology and Ideologies of Western Dominance.* Ithaca, NY: Cornell University Press, 1989.

Albrecht, William. "Soil Fertility and Animal Health: The Albrecht Papers," Vol. 2, second edition. Austin, TX: Acres USA, 2005.

Armour, J. Andrew. *Neurocardiology: Anatomical and Functional Principles.* Boulder, CA: Institute of HeartMath Publications, 2003.

Bateson, Gregory. *Mind and Nature: A Necessary Unity.* New York: E.P. Dutton, 1979.

Beck, Martha. *Expecting Adam: A True Story of Birth, Rebirth, and Everyday Magic.* New York: Times Books, 1999.

Berry, Wendell. *The Unsettling of America: Culture and Agriculture.* San Francisco: Sierra Club Books, 1996.

———. *The Art of the Commonplace: The Agrarian Essays of Wendell Berry.* Berkeley, CA: Counterpoint, 2003.

Bhalla, Jag. *I'm Not Hanging Noodles on Your Ears and Other Intriguing Idioms From Around the World.* Washington, DC: National Geographic, 2009.

Bohm, David. *Wholeness and the Implicate Order.* London: Routledge and Kegan Paul, 1980.

Braden, Gregg. *Awakening to Zero Point: The Collective Initiation,* revised edition. Bellevue, WA: Sacred Spaces and Ancient Wisdom, 1997.

Brezsny, Rob. *Pronoia Is the Antidote for Paranoia: How the Whole World Is Conspiring to Shower You with Blessings,* revised and expanded edition. Berkeley, CA: North Atlantic Books, 2009.

Buhner, Stephen Harrod. *The Lost Language of Plants: The Ecological Importance of Plant Medicines for Life on Earth.* White River Junction, VT: Chelsea Green, 2002.

———. *The Secret Teachings of Plants: In the Direct Perception of Nature.* Rochester, VT: Bear and Company, 2004.

Carlos, Tracie. *Connor's Gift: Embracing Autism in This New Age.* Blissful Heart Publishers (CreateSpace LLC), 2011.

Childre, D., and H. Martin. *The HeartMath Solution.* San Francisco: HarperSanFrancisco, 1999.

Childre, Doc, and Deborah Rozman, PhD. *Transforming Anxiety: The HeartMath® Solution for Overcoming Fear and Worry.* Oakland, CA: New Harbinger Publications, 2006.

Conrad, Ross. *Natural Beekeeping: Organic Approaches to Modern Apiculture.* White River Junction, VT: Chelsea Green, 2007.

Conservation Biology, Vol. 22, No. 6, Society for Conservation Biology. DOI: 10.1111/j.1523-1739.2008.01101.x (2008), pp. 1376–1377.

A Course in Miracles. Mill Valley, CA: The Foundation for Inner Peace, 1975; http://acim.org/.

Damasio, Antonio R. *Descartes' Error: Emotion, Reason and the Human Brain.* New York: Avon Books, 1994.

Darwin, Charles. *The Descent of Man*, second edition, 1871; digireads.com, 2009.

Dyer, Wayne. *Manifest Your Destiny: The Nine Spiritual Principles for Getting Everything You Want.* New York: Harper Paperbacks, 1997.

Emoto, Masaru. *The Hidden Messages in Water.* Hillsboro, OR: Beyond Words Publishing, 2004.

Estrada, Alvaro. *Maria Sabina: Her Life and Chants.* Santa Barbara, CA: Ross Erickson, 1981.

Fallon, Sally. *Nourishing Traditions: The Cookbook that Challenges Politically Correct Nutrition and the Diet Dictocrats*, revised second edition. Washington, DC: New Trends Publishing, 1999.

Findhorn Community. *The Findhorn Garden: Pioneering a New Vision of Humanity and Nature in Cooperation*, third edition. Forres, Scotland: Findhorn Press, 2003.

Gerber, Richard. *Vibrational Medicine: The #1 Handbook of Subtle-Energy Therapies*, third edition. Rochester, VT: Bear & Company, 2001.

Goodall, Jane. *Jane Goodall: 50 Years at Gombe*, first edition. New York:

Stewart, Tabori & Chang, 2010.

Goswami, Amrit, PhD. *The Quantum Doctor: A Physicist's Guide to Health and Healing.* Charlottesville, VA: Hampton Roads, 2004.

Grossinger, Richard. *Embryos, Galaxies, and Sentient Beings: How the Universe Makes Life.* Berkeley, CA: North Atlantic Books, 2003.

———. *Embryogenesis: Species, Gender, and Identity.* Berkeley, CA: North Atlantic Books, 2000.

Hart, Tobin, PhD. *The Secret Spiritual World of Children.* Novato, CA: New World Library, 2003.

Hartmann, Thom. *The Last Hours of Ancient Sunlight.* New York: Three Rivers Press, 1998.

Heisenberg, Werner. *Physics and Philosophy: The Revolution in Modern Science.* New York: Harper and Row, 1962.

Hicks, Esther and Jerry. *Ask and It Is Given: Learning to Manifest Your Desires.* Carlsbad, CA: Hay House, 2004.

———. *The Law of Attraction: The Basics of the Teachings of Abraham.* Carlsbad, CA: Hay House, 2006.

———. *The Vortex: Where the Law of Attraction Assembles All Cooperative Relationships.* Carlsbad, CA: Hay House, 2009.

Holmes, Ernest. *The Science of Mind: A Philosophy, A Faith, A Way of Life.* New York: Tarcher Putnam updated edition, 1998.

Holmgren, David. *Permaculture: Principles and Pathways Beyond Sustainability.* Hepburn, Victoria, Australia: Holmgren Design Services, 2002.

Huff, Darrell. *How to Lie With Statistics.* New York: W.W. Norton, 1954; reissue 1993.

Jackson, Wes. *Becoming Native to This Place.* New York: Counterpoint, 1996.

Jacobsen, Rowan. *Fruitless Fall: The Collapse of the Honeybee and the Coming Agricultural Crisis.* New York: Bloomsbury USA, 2009.

Jenny, Hans. *Cymatics: A Study of Wave Phenomena and Vibration.* Combined Volumes One and Two. Newmarket, NH: Macromedia Publishing, 2001.

Jung, Carl Gustav. *Man and his Symbols.* New York: Dell Publishing, 1968.

———. *Memories, Dreams, Reflections.* New York: Vintage Books, 1962.

Katz, Sandor Ellis. *Wild Fermentation: The Flavor, Nutrition and Craft of Live-Culture Foods.* White River Junction, VT: Chelsea Green, 2003.

Keith, Lierre. *The Vegetarian Myth: Food Justice and Sustainability.* Oakland, CA: PM Press, 2009.

Laszlo, Ervin. *Science and the Akashic Field: An Integral Theory of Everything.* Rochester, VT: Inner Traditions, 2004.

Lauck, Joanne Elizabeth. *The Voice of the Infinite in the Small: Revisioning the Insect-Human Connection.* Boston: Shambhala, 2002.

Lipton, Bruce. *The Biology of Belief: Unleashing the Power of Consciousness, Matter and Miracles.* Santa Rosa, CA: Mountain of Love/Elite Books, 2005.

Logsdon, Gene. *All Flesh is Grass: The Pleasures and Promises of Pasture Farming.* Athens, OH: Swallow Press, 2004.

Lowenfels, Jeff, and Wayne Lewis. *Teaming with Microbes: The Organic Gardener's Guide to the Soil Food Web,* revised edition. Portland, OR: Timber Press, 2010.

Loye, David. *Darwin's Lost Theory of Love: A Healing Vision for the 21st Century.* Lincoln, NE: toExcel, 2000.

———. *Darwin's Lost Theory: Who We Really Are and Where We're Going.* Pacific Grove, CA: Benjamin Franklin Press, 2007.

Maslow, Abraham. *Religions, Values, and Peak-Experiences.* New York: Penguin, 1994.

———. *Toward a Psychology of Being,* third edition. Mansfield Center, CT: Martino, Publishing, 2010.

McTaggert, Lynn. *The Field: The Quest for the Secret Force of the Universe,* updated edition. New York: Harper Paperbacks, 2008.

Monroe, Robert. *Journeys Out of Body,* updated edition. New York: Doubleday, 1992.

———. *Far Journeys.* New York: Doubleday, 1985.

———. *Ultimate Journey.* New York: Three Rivers Press, 1996.

Murray, Maynard. *Sea Energy Agriculture* (reprint). Austin, TX: Acres USA, 2003.

Myss, Caroline, PhD, and C. Norman Shealy, MD, PhD. *The Creation of Health: The Emotional, Psychological, and Spiritual Responses that Promote Health and Healing.* New York: Three Rivers Press, 1988, 1993.

Narby, Jeremy. *The Cosmic Serpent: DNA and the Origins of Knowledge.* New York: Tarcher/Putnam, 1999.

Oschman, James. *Energy Medicine: The Scientific Basis.* Philadelphia: Churchill Livingstone, 2000.

Peace Pilgrim. *Peace Pilgrim: Her Life and Work in Her Own Words.* Santa Fe, NM: Ocean Tree Books, 1982; http://www.peacepilgrim.org/.

Pearce, Joseph Chilton. *The Biology of Transcendence: A Blueprint of the Human Spirit.* Rochester, VT: Park Street Press, 2002.

———. *The Death of Religion and the Rebirth of the Spirit: A Return to the Intelligence of the Heart.* Rochester, VT: Park Street Press, 2007.

Penrose, Roger. *The Large, the Small and the Human Mind.* Cambridge, UK: Cambridge University Press, 2000.

Pert, Candace, PhD. *Molecules of Emotion.* New York: Scribner, 1997.

Pollan, Michael. *The Botany of Desire: A Plant's Eye View of the World.* New York: Random House Trade Paperbacks, 2002.

———. *The Omnivore's Dilemma: A Natural History of Four Meals.* New York: Penguin, 2007.

———. *In Defense of Food: An Eater's Manifesto.* New York: Penguin, 2009.

Prentice, Jessica. *Full Moon Feast: Food and the Hunger for Connection.* White River Junction, VT: Chelsea Green, 2006.

Price, Weston A., DDS. *Nutrition and Physical Degeneration,* eighth edition. La Mesa, CA: Price Pottenger Nutrition, 2008.

Radin, Dean. *The Conscious Universe: The Scientific Truth of Psychic Phenomena.* New York: Harper One, 1997.

———. *Entangled Minds: Extrasensory Experiences in a Quantum Reality.* New York: Paraview Pocket Books, 2006.

Roads, Michael. *Journey Into Nature: A Spiritual Adventure.* Tiburon, CA: HJ Kramer. 1990.

————. *Talking With Nature: Sharing the Energies and Spirit of Trees, Plants, Birds, and Earth*. Tiburon, CA: HJ Kramer, 1997.

Roberts, Jane (Seth) and Robert Butts. *The Individual and the Nature of Mass Events (Seth Book)*. San Rafael, CA: Amber-Allen, 1995.

————. *Seth Speaks: The Eternal Validity of the Soul*. San Rafael, CA: Amber-Allen, 1994.

Ruiz, don Miguel. *The Four Agreements: A Practical Guide to Personal Freedom, A Toltec Wisdom Book*. San Rafael, CA: Amber-Allen, 2001.

Russell, Ronald. *The Journey of Robert Monroe: From Out-of-Body Explorer to Consciousness Pioneer*. Charlottesville, VA: Hampton Roads Publishing, 2007.

Salatin, Joel. *Everything I Want To Do Is Illegal: War Stories From the Local Food Front*. Swoope, VA: Polyface, 2007.

————. *The Sheer Ecstasy of Being a Lunatic Farmer*. Swoope, VA: Polyface, 2010.

Shealy, C. Norman. *90 Days to Stress-Free Living: A Day-by-Day Health Plan Including Exercises, Diet and Relaxation Techniques*. Boston: Element, 1999.

Sheldrake, Rupert. *Dogs That Know When Their Masters are Coming Home and Other Unexplained Powers of Animals*. New York: Three Rivers Press, 1999.

Shiva, Vandana. *Earth Democracy: Justice, Sustainability and Peace*. Cambridge, MA: South End Press, 2005.

————. *Monocultures of the Mind: Perspectives on Biotechnology and Biodiversity*. London: Zed Books, 1993.

Simoncini, T. *Cancer is a Fungus: A Revolution in Tumor Therapy*. Casale Marittimo, Italy: Edizioni Lampis, 2007.

Somé, Malidoma Patrice. *Of Water and The Spirit*. New York: Penguin, 1995.

Stockton, Bayard. *Catapult: The Biography of Robert Monroe*. Norfolk, VA: The Donning Company, 1989.

Szasz, Thomas. *The Second Sin*. London: Routledge and Kegan Paul, 1974.

Talbot, Michael. *The Holographic Universe*. New York: Harper Perennial, first edition, 1992.

Tomkins, Peter, and Christopher Bird. *The Secret Life of Plants: A Fascinating Account of the Physical, Emotional and Spiritual Relations Between Plants and Man.* New York: Harper Paperbacks, 1989.

Voisin, Andre. *Soil, Grass and Cancer: The Link Between Human and Animal Health and the Mineral Balance of the Soil* (reprint). Austin, TX: Acres USA, 2000.

————. *Grass Productivity* (reprint). Washington, DC: Island Press, 1998.

Walters, Charles. *Fertility From the Ocean Deep.* Austin, TX: Acres USA, 2005.

Watts, Alan. *The Book: On the Taboo Against Knowing Who You Are.* New York: Vintage Books, 1989.

————. *Behold the Spirit: A Study in the Necessity of Mystical Religion.* New York: Vintage, 1972.

Williamson, Marianne. *A Return to Love: Reflections on the Principles of "A Course in Miracles."* New York: Harper Paperbacks, 1990.

Wood, Matthew. *The Book of Herbal Wisdom: Using Plants as Medicines.* Berkeley, CA: North Atlantic Books, 1997.

Wright, Machaelle Small. *Behaving as if the God in All Life Mattered,* third revised edition. Warrenton, VA: Perelandra Ltd., 1997.

Films

The Economics of Happiness, www.theeconomicsofhappiness.org
Food, Inc., www.foodincmovie.com
I Am: The Documentary, www.iamthedoc.com

Television

Millan, Cesar. "The Dog Whisperer." The National Geographic Channel
http://channel.nationalgeographic.com/series/dog-whisperer
Cesar Millan's official website: www.cesarsway.com

Audio/Music

Hemi-Sync® can be purchased through the bookstore at the Monroe
Institute or through numerous distributors, bookstores, and music
stores, including my website.
The Monroe Institute: http://www.monroeinstitute.org
Marcey Shapiro: www.marceyshapiro.com

God's Cricket Chorus, a small CD done by Jim Wilson and David Carson, was
originally released in 1992. I was unable to locate any site to purchase
it today, though it seems to be available via various shareware sites.

This American Life, www.thisamericanlife.org
Podcast: www.thisamericanlife.org/podcast

Kate Wolf, www.katewolf.com
A download of the song "Give Yourself to Love" is available through iTunes®.

Organizations and Institutes

The Arlington Institute
www.arlingtoninstitute.org
From their website: "The Arlington Institute is a 501(c)(3) non-profit
research institute that specializes in thinking about global futures and
trying to influence rapid, positive change."

Bioneers: Revolution from the Heart of Nature
www.bioneers.org
A leading-edge forum and annual visionary environmental conference held
annually in San Francisco. Very uplifting! Chock full of inspiring solutions.

Institute of HeartMath®
www.heartmath.org
14700 West Park Ave.
Boulder Creek, CA 95006
Phone: (831) 338-8500 or (800) 711-6221

Institute of Noetic Sciences

    www.noetic.org

    The Institute of Noetic Sciences was founded by *Apollo 14* Astronaut
    Edgar Mitchell after he walked on the moon. IONS' Research and
    Educational Offices are at Foundry Wharf on the Petaluma River in
    downtown Petaluma, California.

River Campus

    Research & Education:
    625 2nd St., Suite 200
    Petaluma, CA 94952-5120

The EarthRise at IONS Retreat Center:

    101 San Antonio Road
    Petaluma, CA 94952

The Land Institute

    www.landinstitute.org

    Researches Natural Systems Agriculture, a mimic of nature's ecosystems.
       Offering programs in education and rural community studies.
    2440 E. Water Well Road
    Salina, KS 67401

The Monroe Institute

    www.monroeinstitute.org
    365 Roberts Mountain Road
    Faber, Virginia 22938
    Phone (434) 361-1252;   Toll-Free (866) 881-3440

Weston A. Price Foundation

    www.westonaprice.org

    From their website: "The Weston A. Price Foundation is a nonprofit,
    tax-exempt charity founded in 1999 to disseminate the research
    of nutrition pioneer Dr. Weston Price, whose studies of isolated
    nonindustrialized peoples established the parameters of human

health and determined the optimum characteristics of human diets."

Periodicals

Christian Science Monitor
>   www.csmonitor.com

Wise Traditions in Food Farming and the Healing Arts
>   www.westonaprice.org/journal-archive
>   Many back issues can be accessed online, but I encourage joining the Weston A. Price Foundation to support their activism.

Atlantis Rising
>   www.atlantisrising.com/index.shtml
>   Quirky but at times visionary look at new technologies, new energy, and history from a novel perspective; extraterrestrials.

FuturEdition
>   TheFuture@FUTUREdition.org
>   Futurist John Petersen's great ezine resource, published weekly, full of information on the future as the present.

Online Resources

Abraham-Hicks, http://Abraham-Hicks.com

Artist Anna Dumitriu and The Normal Flora Project, http://web.mac.com/annadumitriu/NF/Home.html

Australian Bush Flower Remedies, http://ausflowers.com.au

Bach Flower Remedies, www.bachflower.com

Green Hope Farms, www.greenhopeessences.com

HeartMath Institute, www.heartmath.org

Biodynamics of Osteopathy (James Jealous, DO), www.jamesjealous.com

The Monroe Institute, www.monroeinstitute.org

Nova, www.pbs.org/wgbh/nova

Orin and Daben, www.orindaben.com

Society of Ortho-Bionomy® International, http://ortho-bionomy.org

Upledger Institute, www.upledger.com

Weston A. Price Foundation, www.westonaprice.org

The Windbridge Institute, www.windbridge.org

Notes

❦

INTRODUCTION

[1] Wikipedia: Max Planck.

[2] http://quitsmoking.about.com/cs/nicotineinhaler/a/cigingredients.htm.

[3] http://www.epa.gov/radtown/tobacco.html. The Environmental Protection Agency acknowledges that over time radiation in cigarettes and cigarette smoke results in a significant amount of irradiation of the lungs. In fact, in 1990 the surgeon general C. Everett Koop admitted on a nationally televised spot that probably 90% of cancers caused from cigarettes are a result of radiation exposure. It is interesting to note that radiation is found in cigarettes because of chemical-intensive fertilization processes that actually add it to the soil in which tobacco is grown. Organic tobacco would not, by law, have these same additives, so is likely to be free of radioactive contamination. See also www.acsa.net/HealthAlert/radioactive_tobacco.html.

[4] Wigner, Eugene, as quoted in *Remarks on the Mind-Body Question*, in Wheeler and Zurek, *Quantum Theory and Measurement* (p. 169); found in www.informationphilosopher.com/solutions/scientists/ wigner/.

CHAPTER ONE

[1] Heart Embryology, http://pie.med.utoronto.ca/htbg/HTBG_content/ HTBG_heartEmbryologyApp.html.

[2] Joseph Chilton Pearce, *The Biology of Transcendence: A Blueprint of the Human Spirit* (Rochester, VT: Park Street Press, 2002), p. 56.

[3] Rollin McCraty, "The Energetic Heart: Bioelectromagnetic Communication Within and Between People," chapter published in: *Clinical Applications of Bioelectromagnetic Medicine*. Edited by P.J. Rosch and M.S. Markov (New York: Marcel Dekker, 2004), pp. 541–562.

[4] Joseph Chilton Pearce, *The Death of Religion and the Rebirth of the Spirit* (Rochester, VT: Park Street Press, 2007), p. 67.

[5] D. Childre and H. Martin, *The HeartMath Solution* (San Francisco: Harper-SanFrancisco, 1999), pp. 158–161.

[6] In rereading *The HeartMath Solution* after writing this book (to look for half-remembered quotes), I realized that many of their concepts influenced my book, especially the introduction and first chapter. I initially read *The HeartMath Solution* shortly after it was published in 1999, and I see now that it had a seminal effect upon my thinking. I am deeply indebted to their pioneering research and thought.

[7] Rollin McCraty, Mike Atkinson, and Raymond T. Bradley, "Electrophysiological Evidence of Intuition. Part 1: The Surprising Role of the Heart," *Journal of Alternative and Complementary Medicine* 10(1) (2004), pp. 133–143.

[8] Lorenzo Langstroth, as quoted in http://sites.google.com/site/mikelenehan/theessenceofbeeing, from Langstroth's 1853 book *The Hive and the Honey Bee*.

[9] Joseph Chilton Pearce, *The Biology of Transcendence*, p. 56.

CHAPTER TWO

[1] *Technology Review*, www.technologyreview.com/communications/37357/?a=f.

[2] No Sweat Shakespeare, www.nosweatshakespeare.com/resources/shakespeare-words.htm.

[3] Karl Albrecht in Famous Quotes://thinkexist.com/quotes/karl_albrecht/.

[4] www.1-famous-quotes.com/quote/1361084.

[5] The tool I am referring to here is the emotional scale, detailed in the book *Ask and It Is Given*. By noting where one is emotionally it is easier to move to a better-feeling place, and by making this shift to create a more desired life outcome.

The Abraham-Hicks website offers a number of explanations of who Abraham is, and how Esther Hicks translates their wisdom into her words. Look under the heading "About Abraham-Hicks" to find several descriptions including: "Abraham has described themselves as 'a group consciousness from the non-physical dimension'" (which helps a lot!). They have also said, "We are that which you are. You are the leading edge of that which we are. We are that which is at the heart of all religions." The teachings offer practical tools for improving life based on principles acknowledging the Law of Attraction. They are not a religion or a religious-affiliated organization. The teachings of Abraham are available in an array of formats, including books, CDs, and live workshops. The URL for their website is: www.abraham-hicks.com/lawofattractionsource/index.php. If you are intrigued by their ideas, note that they have an excellent (in my opinion) full-length introductory CD available as a free download.

CHAPTER THREE

[1] *The Free Online Dictionary,* www.thefreedictionary.com/premises.

[2] Dictionary.com; http://dictionary.reference.com/browse/premise.

[3] *Journal of the Royal Society of Medicine,* Vol. 94, No. 9 (September 2001): pp. 458–461; www.ncbi.nlm.nih.gov/pmc/articles/PMC1282187/.

[4] Ulrike Bingel, Vishvarani Wanigasekera, Katja Wiech, Roisin Ni Mhuircheartaigh, Michael C. Lee, Markus Ploner, and Irene Tracey, "The Effect of Treatment Expectation on Drug Efficacy: Imaging the Analgesic Benefit of the Opioid Remifentanil," *Science Translational Medicine* (16 February 2011), 3:70ra14.

And see commentary by Mike Adams, www.naturalnews.com/031451_drug_trials_placebo_effect.html#ixzz1EwGZZZsQ.

[5] Christopher Peterson, Martin E. Seligman, George E. Vaillant, "Pessimistic explanatory style is a risk factor for physical illness: A thirty-five-year longitudinal study," *Journal of Personality and Social Psychology,* Vol. 55, No. 1 (July 1988): pp. 23–27.

[6] *Harvard Men's Health Watch* (May 2008); www.health.harvard.edu/
press_releases/why-optimists-enjoy-better-health.

[7] U.S. Department of Health and Human Services, National Health Expenditure Factsheet 2009, www.cms.gov/NationalHealthExpendData/25_NHE_Fact_Sheet.asp.

[8] http://en.wikipedia.org/wiki/Military_budget_of_the_United_States.

[9] http://updates.pain-topics.org/2010/03/nsaid-dangers-may-limit-pain-relief.html.

From GI bleeding alone there are at least 16,500 deaths with 120,000 hospitalizations annually. There is also significant increased risk of stroke, heart attack, and damage to kidneys from NSAIDs, so total deaths secondary to NSAIDs is widely estimated at 30,000 annually in the U.S. See also *Journal of the American Medical Association*, Vol. 286 (August 22/29 2001): pp. 954–959.

AIDS death statistics: www.avert.org/usa-statistics.htm; currently in the U.S. there are 16,000 to 18,000 AIDS deaths per year.

[10] LeeAnne Harker and Dacher Keltner, University of California, Berkeley, "Expressions of Positive Emotion in Women's College Yearbook Pictures and Their Relationship to Personality and Life Outcomes Across Adulthood,"
http://education.ucsb.edu/janeconoley/ed197/documents/Keltnerexpressionsofpositivemotion.pdf.

[11] John C. Barefoot, Beverly H. Brummett, Redford B. Williams, Ilene C. Siegler, Michael J. Helms, Stephen H. Boyle, Nancy E. Clapp-Channing, and Daniel B. Mark, "Recovery Expectations and Long-term Prognosis of Patients With Coronary Heart Disease," *Archive of Internal Medicine* (February 2011): pp. 411–417.

[12] Ernest Abel and Michael Kruger, "Smile Intensity in Photographs Predicts Longevity," *Psychological Science* (February 26, 2010).

[13] National Institutes of Health: Hydrocephalus, www.nlm.nih.gov/medlineplus/ency/article/001571.htm.

[14] "Das Wesen der Materie" (The Nature of Matter), speech at Florence, Italy, 1944 (from Archiv zur Geschichte der Max-Planck-Gesellschaft, Abt. Va, Rep. 11 Planck, Nr. 1797).

[15] www.brainyquote.com/quotes/authors/p/pierre_teilhard_de_chardin. html.

Chapter Four

No notes

Chapter Five

[1] www.brainyquote.com/quotes/authors/a/alan_watts.html.

[2] www.timesonline.co.uk/tol/news/science/article6539405.ece.

[3] Dean Radin, PhD, *The Conscious Universe* (New York: Harper Collins, 1997), pp. 161–169.

[4] Masaru Emoto, *The Hidden Messages in Water* (Hillsboro, OR: Beyond Words Publishing, 2004).

[5] http://en.wikipedia.org/wiki/Gut_flora.

[6] Kenneth Todar, PhD, "Normal Flora" in *Todar's Online Textbook of Bacteriology;* www.textbookofbacteriology.net/index.html.

[7] Medical Microbiology syllabus. Southern Illinois University at Carbondale, 2011; www.cehs.siu.edu/fix/medmicro/normal.htm.

[8] Artist Anna Dumitriu and The Normal Flora Project: http://web.mac.com/annadumitriu/NF/Home.html.

Chapter Six

[1] *This American Life* podcast: www.thisamericanlife.org/podcast.

[2] Vilayanur Ramachandran: "The Neurons that Shaped Civilization," TedIndia2009 (posted online January 2010); www.ted.com/talks/vs_ramachandran_the_neurons_that_shaped_civilization.html.

[3] Dean Radin, PhD, "The Global Consciousness Project," in *Entangled Minds* (New York: Paraview Pocket Books, 2006), pp. 195–207.

Chapter Seven

[1] Antonia Fraser, *King Charles II* (New Haven, CT: Phoenix Press, 2007).

[2] PB Wood Methodology and Apologetics: Thomas Sprat's "History of the Royal Society," *The British Journal for the History of Science*, Vol. 13, No. 1 (March 1980): pp. 1–26.

[3] Ed. Jack Lynch. Sprat, Thomas, *History of the Royal Society*, 1667. For selections see http://ethnicity.rutgers.edu/~jlynch/Texts/sprat.html and Don Watson, *The Religion of Scientism*, www.enformy.com/Religion_of_Scientism.htm.

[4] Ibid. Jack Lynch.

[5] Rupert Sheldrake, *Dogs That Know When Their Masters are Coming Home and Other Unexplained Powers of Animals* (New York: Three Rivers Press, 1999).

[6] M.R. Sadigh, PhD (Director of Psychology, The Gateway Institute) and P.W. Kozicky, MD (Founder and Director, The Gateway Institute), "The Effects of Hemi-Sync on Electrocortical Activity," www.monroe-institute.org/wiki/index.php/The_Effects_of_Hemi-Sync_on_Electro-cortical_Activity#Subject_and_Procedures.

[7] Abraham Maslow, *Religions, Values, and Peak-Experiences* (New York: Penguin, 1994) and Joseph Chilton Pearce, *The Death of Religion and the Rebirth of the Spirit: A Return to the Intelligence of the Heart* (Rochester, VT: Park Street Press, 2007).

Chapter Eight

[1] Charles Darwin, *The Descent of Man*, second edition, 1871; digireads.com, 2009, p. 163.

[2] Geoff Olson, *Kropotkin versus Darwin—Cooperation as an Evolutionary Force;* www.commonground.ca/iss/0509170/cg170_geoff.shtml.

[3] University of Exeter (March 29, 2011), "Evolution: Not only the fittest survive," *ScienceDaily*. Retrieved May 7, 2011, from www.sciencedaily.com/releases/2011/03/110327191044.htm.

4 http://andrewsullivan.thedailybeast.com/2011/04/quote-for-the-day-1.
html.

CHAPTER NINE

1 *Merriam-Webster Open Dictionary*, www.merriam-webster.com/
dictionary/virus.
2 "Genetically Modified Cows Produce Human Milk," *The Telegraph* (May
8, 2011); www.telegraph.co.uk/earth/agriculture/geneticmodifica-
tion/8423536/Genetically-modified-cows-produce-human-milk.html.
3 Purdue University Professor Emeritus of Plant Physiology, Dr. Don Huber, petitioned Tom Vilsack of the USDA to postpone approval of GM
Alfalfa, based upon his research showing a novel and deadly organism
infecting animals who consume those crops. The organism affects humans as well as horses, pigs, cattle, and poultry, and can kill a fertilized
egg in 24–48 hours. He is interviewed here, discussing his findings:
http://vimeo.com/22997532.

Another article, on the CBS online network bnet, also presents
Dr. Huber's findings: www.bnet.com/blog/food-industry/mystery-
science-more-details-on-the-strange-organism-that-could-destroy-
monsanto/3052.

Nonetheless, Vilsack approved GMO Alfalfa without restrictions as
to where it could be planted.
4 Organic Consumers Association, www.organicconsumers.org/articles/
article_22625.cfm.
5 Discovery News (June 2010); http://news.discovery.com/space/the-
higgs-boson-may-have-five-faces.html.

CHAPTER TEN

1 I originally read this study I describe when I was in medical school and it
struck me deeply, but I could not find the original reference later. Still,
there is a lot of information on immune effects of racism. The article
"Racism is Unhealthy, Literally," which aired on NPR's *Tell Me More*

on February 15, 2010, goes into detail about many recent studies that
have been done examining the detrimental immune effects of racism;
www.npr.org/templates/story/story.php?storyId=123668467.

² Max Planck in Wikiquotes; http://en.wikiquote.org/wiki/Max_Planck.

³ Centers for Disease Control and Prevention: Investigation Announce-
ment: Multistate Outbreak of E. coli O157:H7 Infections Associated
with Lebanon Bologna; www.cdc.gov/ecoli/.

⁴ Marler Clark law firm; www.about-ecoli.com/.

⁵ Associated Press on MSNBC about the Topps meat closure in 2007: 21.7
million pounds of ground beef, representing an entire year's production, were eventually recalled due to contamination. The related law-
suits are still in the court system. www.msnbc.msn.com/id/21149977/.

⁶ *Christian Science Monitor Online:* www.csmonitor.com/Busi-
ness/new-economy/2010/0819/Egg-recall-list-expands.-
Check-your-eggs-again. See also Marler Clark Law Firm
Food Safety News, www.foodsafetynews.com/2011/02/
fda-finds-salmonella-in-first-round-of-egg-facility-testing/.

⁷ I was inspired, in writing this chapter, by articles in *Wise Traditions*
magazine, several of the works of Joel Salatin, and Jessica Prentice's
wonderful *Full Moon Feast: Food and the Hunger for Connection,* and I
gratefully acknowledge their contributions to my thought and writing.

CHAPTER ELEVEN

¹ Paul Stamets, "Fungi and the Ecosystem," www.fungi.com/mycotech/
mycova.html.

² Oregon Sustainable Agriculture Land Trust, January 1996.

³ IAASTD, "Agriculture at a Crossroads,"
www.agassessment.org/reports/IAASTD/EN/Agriculture%20at%20
a%20Crossroads_Global%20Report%20(English).pdf.

⁴ K. Edwards and C. Zierholz, "Soil formation and erosion rates." In: *Soils:
Their Properties and Management* (Eds. P.E.V. Charman and B.W. Mur-
phy), second edition (Oxford University Press, 2000), pp. 39–58.

[5] "Soil Carbon" from the Soil Association, www.soilassociation.org/Whyorganic/Climatefriendlyfoodandfarming/Soilcarbon/tabid/574/Default.aspx.

[6] www.soilassociation.org/

[7] Polyface Farms, www.polyfacefarms.com/.

[8] IAASTD, "Agriculture at a Crossroads" (see note 3 above).

[9] Ibid., p. 540.

[10] Allan Savory and others, "Moving the World Toward Sustainability," *Green Money Journal*, www.greenmoney.com. As quoted in *Wise Traditions*, "An Inconvenient Cow" (May 2009); www.westonaprice.org/farm-a-ranch/1639-an-inconvenient-cow.

[11] Paul Stamets, *Fungi Perfecti*, "The Petroleum Problem," www.fungi.com/mycotech/petroleum_problem.html.

[12] A PubMed search returns 2426 abstracts referencing fungus in cancer patients. One interesting study is this one, from Mexico. It showed increasingly more virulent species in patients the more advanced their cancers. *Revista Latinoamericana de Microbiologia*, Vol. 40, Nos. 1-2 (Jan-June 1998): pp. 15–24.

For another discussion on fungal agents isolated from cancer patients, see:

Alvarez Gasca MA, Argüero Licea B., Pliego Castañeda A., García Tena S.,

www.ncbi.nlm.nih.gov/pubmed/10932730.

CHAPTER TWELVE

[1] Dean Radin, PhD, *The Conscious Universe* (New York: Harper Collins, 1997).

[2] Thomas Szasz, *The Second Sin* (London: Routledge and Kegan Paul, 1974).

[3] Darrell Huff, *How to Lie With Statistics* (New York: W.W. Norton, 1954, reissue 1993), p. 8.

CHAPTER THIRTEEN

[1] World Research Foundation, "The Power of Mind and the Promise of Placebo," www.wrf.org/alternative-therapies/power-of-mind-placebo.php.

[2] Bruce Moseley, MD, et al., "A Controlled Trial of Arthroscopic Surgery for Osteoarthritis of the Knee," *The New England Journal of Medicine*, Vol. 347 (July 11 2002): pp. 81–88.

[3] My father, Robert Shapiro, a wise and loving parent who influenced me throughout my life, passed away during the editing phase of this book, so is no longer on any medications and is instead blissfully supporting me from the other side. After consideration I chose to leave references to him unchanged in the final manuscript and added this endnote.

[4] Barbara Starfield, MD, MPH, "Is US Health Really the Best in the World?", *Journal of the American Medical Association* or *JAMA*, Vol. 284, No. 4 (July 26, 2000), p. 483; http://jama.amaassn.org/content/284/4/483.extract and www.avaresearch.com/avamainwebsite/files/20100401061256.pdf?page=files/20100401061256.pdf.

[5] www.car-accidents.com/pages/stats.html.

[6] Gary Null, PhD, Carolyn Dean, MD ND, Martin Feldman, MD, Debora Rasio, MD, and Dorothy Smith, PhD, "The American Medical System is the Leading Cause of Death and Injury in the United States," www.webdc.com/pdfs/deathbymedicine.pdf.

CHAPTER FOURTEEN

No notes

CHAPTER FIFTEEN

[1] *The Early Show*, 2006, "How a Blind Teen 'Sees' with Sound," www.cbsnews.com/stories/2006/07/19/earlyshow/main1817689.shtml.

[2] Bayard Stockton, *Catapult: The Biography of Robert Monroe* (Norfolk, VA: The Donning Company, 1989).

[3] Ronald Russell, *The Journey of Robert Monroe: From Out-of-Body Explorer to Consciousness Pioneer* (Charlottesville, VA: Hampton Roads Publishing, 2007).

CHAPTER SIXTEEN

[1] Werner Heisenberg, *Physics and Philosophy: The Revolution in Modern Science* (New York: Harper and Row, 1962).

[2] Science News online edition, www.sciencenews.org/view/generic/id/72302/title/Fermilab_data_hint_at_possible_new_particle.

[3] http://techie-buzz.com/science/eureka-moment-new-particle-discovered-at-tevatron.html.

[4] Quoted from Dean Radin, *Entangled Minds* (New York: Paraview Pocket Books, 2006). Original citation: Bernard D'Espangnat, "The Quantum Theory and Reality," in *Scientific American* (November 1979): pp. 158–181.

[5] www.bbc.co.uk/programmes/b00xxgbn. The program itself is not currently available, but selections from it are found on YouTube.

[6] Roger Penrose, *The Large, the Small and the Human Mind* (Cambridge, England: Cambridge University Press, 2000), p. 66.

[7] The allegory of the cave is found in Book Seven of *The Republic*. The website called "The History Guide: Lectures on Modern European Intellectual History" contains a good translation of the entire dialogue: www.historyguide.org/intellect/allegory.html.

[8] There is a great deal of data available on this simple, natural, sustainable, and healthy method of nourishing the soil. There is simply no need for chemical fertilizers. Maynard Murray was a visionary medical doctor and soil scientist who looked at the importance of minerals for human health. His original work has been recently reprinted, and the founder of Acres USA, Charles Walters, has continued to expand Murray's message with his own work.

Maynard Murray, *Sea Energy Agriculture* (reprint) (Austin, TX: Acres USA), 2003; and Charles Walters, *Fertility From the Ocean Deep* (Acres USA, 2005).

[9] www.technewsworld.com/story/Cold-Fusion-It-May-Not-Be-Madness-71916.html?wlc=1306099010.

[10] "Italian Cold Fusion Saga Continues with New Papers Released" (January 2011), http://pesn.com/2011/01/27/9501752_Italian_cold_fusion_saga_continues_with_new_papers_released/.

[11] There are many references that confirm this finding. Here are a few online ones (older), and the numbers are expanding.

From 2004: "Use of Complementary and Alternative Medicine Among American Women," *Women's Health Issues* 15 (2005), pp. 5–13.

Dawn M. Upchurch, PhD, and Laura Chyu, MA, found online at www.hawaii.edu/hivandaids/Use_of_Complementary_and_Alternative_Medicine_Among_American_Women.pdf.

BMC Complementary and Alternative Medicine. Health care utilization among complementary and alternative medicine users in a large military cohort: Martin R. White et al., a study published April 2011 indicating that among military personnel, about 45% of those seeking health care utilized CAM; www.biomedcentral.com/1472-6882/11/27.

E. Ernst, "Prevalence of use of complementary/alternative medicine: a systematic review," *Bulletin of the World Health Organization*, Vol. 78, No. 2 (2000). Prevalence of use of complementary/alternative medicine ranged from 9% to 65%. www.who.int/bulletin/archives/78(2)252.pdf.

[12] Ibid.

Acknowledgments

I T TAKES A VILLAGE TO complete a manuscript. My village includes my many dear friends and loved ones. I appreciate the many contributions and rich support of my beloved community.

Star Woodward, the best partner and spouse in the world, read the manuscript over and over, helping me at every stage. She gave me insights, clarified my perceptions, and challenged me to remain uplifting even when the issues were still active for me. She also supported me with extra loads of laundry, sink-fulls of washed dishes, dog walks, spot shoulder massages, Ortho-Bionomy® treatments, and general life maintenance. I adore her!

Julie Klenn is an amazing friend, volunteer editor, and massage therapist. She understands what I am saying and cuts through overly flowery and bulky language to reveal the heart. I have utilized much of her well-tempered advice. Mary Selna, your enthusiasm and supportive comments on the manuscript buoyed me. Bonnie Netherton, your technical editing was spot-on. Susan Benson, your whole approach to life is inspiring, and I loved your occasional comments and unflagging support. Miklane Janner, you are a great friend and so gentle at pointing out some of my more odious word repetitions. I thank Mike and Karen Sherlock for their support, friendship, and encouragement in getting me to focus on writing one book at a time.

I resoundingly acknowledge my heartfelt appreciation for Esther and Jerry Hicks and the Abraham teachings. They live by the clarity of their wonderful example. Their words and teachings have become interwoven in my medical practice and the ways I live my daily life. Their wisdom is reflected throughout this volume. I appreciate as well the many fine folks associated with them who I have met through their seminars and cruises especially Robert Golden, who wrote the foreword, and his spouse Carol Carpenter.

Many other spiritual teachers have influenced me: Seth/Jane Roberts and Robert Butts, and Sanaya Roman and Duane Packer for the Orin and Daben work, especially the lovely Orin guided meditations, which have often lifted me from the doldrums of life. I am deeply influenced by my Jewish heritage, its mysticism and liturgy and its respect for the cycles of life. I appreciate the influence of my early teachers, especially Daniel Matt, my first Kabbalah instructor, and Rabbi Zalman-Schachter-Shalomi and the help he gave me in shaping my thought. I also want to thank the many other wonderful spiritual teachers, living and dead, who publish and write from their visions and clarity: including Marianne Williamson, Alice Walker, Wayne Dyer, Deepak Chopra, Alan Watts, Paramahamsa Yogananda, Meher Baba, Ramana Maharshi, J. Krishnamurti, Ram Dass, and the spiritual wisdom that has passed down through the ages in mystical thought of all traditions.

I am perennially appreciative of everyone associated with the Monroe Institute: the founder, Robert Monroe, for his vision; Laurie Monroe who actualized and expanded upon it; Paul Rademacher, the current Executive Director; Skip Atwater, the president and the individual who has gently supported me during many prep sessions; and all the amazing residential trainers I have worked with—Karen Malik, Patty Ray Avalon, Penny Holmes, Carol Sabick, John Kortum, Lee Stone, and Joe Gallenberger, with a super special thanks to Franceen King for developing and guiding the amazing Starlines programs. You have all expanded my horizons and perceptions. Many areas of great flow in this book are a testament to power of the Hemi-Sync creativity CDs.

I thank my parents for always believing in me, even if they did not always understand me. They are passionate, loving, good, and honorable people. I deeply appreciate the extra boost my dad has sent me from the other side since his death during the final revisions of this book.

I also thank two of my sweet muses, Sean Shapiro and Jasper Hamilton, for the delightfully frank perspective that only two-year-olds can offer. I acknowledge the sustaining grace, humor, and magic of my wonderful and loving friends and family.

I deeply appreciate everyone I have worked with from the professional staff at North Atlantic Books. We have had an outstanding working relationship throughout the process of writing and editing the book. I especially want to thank Richard Grossinger for believing in me and gently urging me to publish, as well as for our ongoing medical/spiritual dialogue; Doug Reil for his vision and perspective; Emily Boyd for her clarity and accessibility; and my professional editor Kathy Glass, who I think is amazing! She sees every nuance of punctuation and flow, really understands the spirit of my book, and has helped me to further craft it. I also want to give a hearty thank-you to Susan Quasha for her lovely cover art. It is exactly what I hoped for.

Thanks to my office staff, also dear friends, for organizing the flow in my life so well, giving me space and clarity for writing: Morgyne Le Count, Julia Goerlitz, Dominique Banuelos, Kate, Rini, and Florena Shapiro.

Finally I thank Nature herself and the clear communications I have enjoyed my entire life. I thank the great variety of microbes, the songbirds, the pink-flowered rhododendron, and profusion of roses outside my bedroom window, the ever-changing five-acre natural area blocks from my home, and the original owners of my house who lovingly planted and tended the inspiring garden. I thank clouds, trees, and God/source/spirit for this amazing world.

About the Author

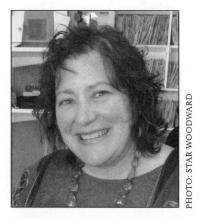

M ARCEY SHAPIRO, MD, IS A family physician who has extensive training and experience in many areas of natural medicine, including Western and Chinese herbal medicine, acupuncture, mind-body techniques, flower essences, homeopathy, breathing techniques, nutritional therapies, and Scenar®, and hands-on modalities such as Ortho-Bionomy® and Biodynamic Osteopathy. Her approach to care is patient-centered and participatory. Dr. Shapiro works with patients to address the many facets of illness/imbalance—biophysical, psychological, and spiritual—and creates realistic treatment plans that incorporate a variety of modalities. Visit her website at:

www.marceyshapiromd.com